Responsible Research Conduct

I0875874

Over 30,000 research articles have been retracted from peer-reviewed journals in recent years, exposing a troubling crisis in research integrity. Beneath this visible tip of the iceberg lies a vast, hidden burden of flawed research, with many cases of misconduct remaining undisclosed or inadequately addressed, while leading institutions have faced allegations of research misconduct, shaking public trust in science.

Confronting the growing disillusionment with unethical practices in research and in the publication of research findings, this book critically examines publicly available reports from institutions, journals, regulators, courts, and platforms like PubPeer and academic blogs, shedding light on systemic failures and the lack of transparency in addressing misconduct. By consolidating lessons from these cases, it offers practical strategies to prevent fraud, improve research practices, and restore trust in the scientific process.

Key Features:

- Offers a comprehensive analysis of research misconduct investigation reports, highlighting systemic issues and root causes.
- Provides actionable lessons for individuals and organizations to improve research practices and uphold integrity.
- Recommends targeted strategies for preventing misconduct and correcting the scientific record post-incident.

Essential for researchers, clinicians, journal editors, academic publishers, funders, and anyone involved in health research, this book provides a roadmap for fostering accountability and integrity in science. Through objective analysis and actionable recommendations, it inspires a more optimistic outlook for the future of research.

Responsible Research Conduct

WHAT INVESTIGATIONS INTO ALLEGED RESEARCH MISCONDUCT TELL US ABOUT SCIENTIFIC INTEGRITY

Khalid S. Khan

CRC Press
Taylor & Francis Group
Boca Raton London New York

CRC Press is an imprint of the
Taylor & Francis Group, an **informa** business

Designed cover image: Shutterstock

First edition published 2026
by CRC Press
2385 NW Executive Center Drive, Suite 320, Boca Raton FL 33431

and by CRC Press
4 Park Square, Milton Park, Abingdon, Oxon, OX14 4RN

CRC Press is an imprint of Taylor & Francis Group, LLC

ISBN: 9781041106036 (hbk)
ISBN: 9781041106029 (pbk)
ISBN: 9781003655916 (ebk)

DOI: 10.1201/9781003655916

Typeset in Minion
by Deanta Global Publishing Services, Chennai, India

Contents

Preface

The first half of this decade witnessed over 30,000 retractions of articles from peer-reviewed research journals. These numbers are staggering and shocking from both professional and lay public perspectives. Society expects academic institutions to uphold the highest standards of research integrity. Yet top universities such as Harvard, Stanford, University College London, Karolinska, and others have been implicated in scandals involving allegations of research misconduct.

There remains a substantial burden of flawed research below the surface. The iceberg of integrity failures reveals retractions at its tip, while the bulk of the defects remains hidden in its submerged portion. Lately, as post-publication peer review has taken an independent form on online platforms such as PubPeer and academic blogs, many research integrity concerns and allegations have become public. By contrast, the investigations into the allegations themselves have largely remained secret. Hence, the ability to conduct any form of root cause analysis has been limited. Where transparency requirements have led to public disclosures of investigation reports by institutions, journals, regulators, courts, and other bodies, awareness of the depth of irresponsible research and publication has been heightened. A critical appraisal of the findings documented in these disclosures also presents a learning opportunity. This book consolidates lessons learned from case studies of a sample of research misconduct investigations to develop fraud prevention strategies and improve research integrity.

There is a need to address the growing disillusionment and cynicism about unethical and unprofessional practices by researchers, academic institutions, publishers, funders, and other stakeholders. Healthy skepticism, grounded in objective analysis of publicly available investigation reports, can lead to a more optimistic outlook.

Khalid S. Khan
2026

About the author

Khalid S. Khan is Professor of Public Health and Preventive Medicine at the University of Granada, Spain. He has been Distinguished Investigator of the prestigious Beatriz Galindo program of the Spanish Ministry of Education, Professor at the University of Birmingham and Queen Mary University of London, UK, and Spinoza Professor at the University of Amsterdam, the Netherlands. His research expertise was recognized in his appointment as a Senior Investigator of the UK National Institute of Health Research. He was the founding Director of the WHO Collaborating Centers for Research in Birmingham and London, UK. He has won several prestigious awards, including the Sims Black Fellowship of the Royal College of Obstetricians and Gynaecologists and the Strutt and Harper Grant of the British Medical Association, UK.

He has covered the complete range of patient-oriented research in his career spanning three decades. As a journal editor, he has presided over 10,000 manuscript evaluations. As a scientific author, he has over 600 publications in peer-reviewed research journals. In his role as director of research and development, he has had the responsibility for providing a governance framework for health research. He has undertaken investigations of allegations of scientific misconduct among studies in progress and post-publication. He has led an international initiative to generate multi-stakeholder consensus on the integrity of clinical trials. He has been a member of grant-giving panels for assessing and awarding trials in the UK and Germany. Supervision of study conduct and analysis, independent oversight and data monitoring, and evidence synthesis and guidelines have all been part of his experience. None of his published studies has been subjected to retraction. He has supervised doctoral students and has examined doctoral theses in Denmark, the Netherlands, Spain, and the UK. With an *h*-index >100, his work has attracted a high level of citations. He has been ranked consistently amongst the top 2% of the world's most influential scientists.Over the last five years, he has meticulously searched and collated several of the reports of research misconduct investigations made public. In some cases, there are multiple investigations of the same integrity concerns. Through this book, he targets specific research integrity concerns, providing updated recommendations for research integrity guidelines.

Acknowledgments

I extend my sincere thanks to Professor Aurora Bueno-Cavanillas from the Department of Public Health and Preventive Medicine at the University of Granada, Spain, for her valuable critical reviews of the early drafts of the book's chapters.

Disclaimer

This book discusses publicly available scientific literature, documents, reports, judgments, testimonies, and correspondence in the context of research integrity. It is intended for educational and scholarly purposes only and does not allege research misconduct, fraud, or intentional wrongdoing by any party. The investigations or proceedings included in the book and the related discussion reflect the publicly available information at the time of writing this book and do not imply any final determination. References to organizations or institutions are made solely in the context of publicly reported cases and do not imply culpability. All statements regarding potential questionable research or publication practices are presented as analysis or opinion based on cited sources and should not be construed as factual assertions of fault. Readers are encouraged to consult the primary sources and form their own conclusions.

Abbreviations

ALLEA	ALL European Academies
CoARA	Coalition for Advancing Research Assessment
COPE	Committee on Publication Ethics
DORA	Declaration on Research Assessment
ICMJE	International Committee of Medical Journal Editors
SCOPE	Start with what is valued, Context considerations, Options for evaluating, Probe deeply, and Evaluate the evaluation
TOP	Transparency and Openness Promotion guidelines
WAME	World Association of Medical Editors

1 *Introduction*

Scientists hold a prestigious position in society, as their work builds expectations of tangible benefits from innovation and discoveries. However, trust in science has been undermined by recent high-profile fraud scandals. To address this, an explicit commitment to research ethics and professionalism is crucial, requiring greater accountability from scientists and the stakeholder organizations that engage in research and publication. Organizational culture strongly influences the behavior of scientists. When research integrity policies and procedures are in place, and adherence to research regulations is valued, there is a good chance that scientists will be able to exercise intellectual honesty without fear. On the other hand, if research integrity principles and standards are routinely flouted and this irresponsible behavior is tolerated without anyone batting an eye, there will be no hesitation in taking up opportunities to manipulate the design, conduct, analysis, or reporting of research to achieve particular outcomes. Investigations of research misconduct allegations and questionable practices shed light on these deficiencies. They offer insight into how organizations fail to safeguard research and publication integrity, and what can be done for better protection. This book takes a deep dive into responsible conduct in research and publication, examining publicly available reports, investigations, court judgments, and expert testimonies to determine the root causes and learn lessons.

Research integrity: Undertaking research following ethical and professional principles and standards. Responsible research and publication practices pave the way for science to be regarded as trustworthy. Integrity failures may result from honest errors or deliberate misconduct.

Retraction: Removing a published paper from the research record due, for example, to the discovery of a flaw in its integrity.

Responsible research and publication

The dreaded words "retraction" and "expression of concern" are on the rise in the published research literature. The graph looks like a tsunami, metaphorically representing a gigantic wave of research fraud, misconduct, and questionable practices that has emerged in the scientific ocean and has hit the coast where public trust resided (Box 1.1). In the PubMed database, there were around 30,000 retractions in 2021–24, whereas just a couple of decades earlier, there were only a few retractions annually. During the same period, there were around 2000 expressions of concern. PubMed is a free-to-access biomedical research database that contains records of articles published in around 5000 journals covering health-related subjects. The total number of retractions and expressions of concern is likely to be much higher in health, biomedicine, and life sciences research, as an estimated 16,000 journals exist in this domain, according to the Science, Technology and Medicine (STM) publishers report.

Expression of concern: A note published by a journal to inform readers of there being the possibility of a concern about the integrity of a paper.

PubMed: A freely available interface of the general biomedical research database Medline.

DOI: 10.1201/9781003655916-1

Box 1.1 Terminology and trends in correction of the scientific record

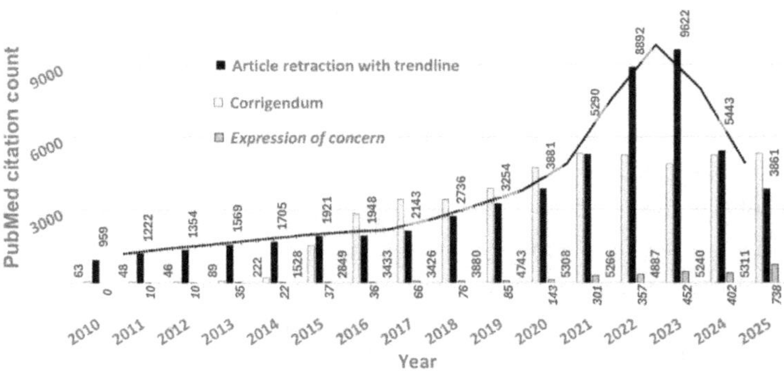

The terminology *(this is a brief overview; see Glossary for details)*

- **Research integrity:** Responsible research and publication in accordance with ethical and professional principles and standards.
- **Version of record:** The final published version of a paper (following peer review, editorial assessments, and author revisions of the manuscript submitted) in its definitive form with copyediting and typesetting completed, metadata applied, and DOI (digital object identifier) allocated.
- **Preprint:** A publicly posted draft version of a scientific manuscript before completion of its formal peer review by a journal. It is usually posted at the first submission of the manuscript to a journal.
- **Expression of concern:** A note published by a journal to inform readers of a possible integrity concern about a published paper.
- **Retraction:** Removal of a published article from the scientific record because of a variety of reasons, including the discovery of a flaw in its integrity, e.g., a post-publication reassessment showing that the data or results reported have major errors. A research misconduct investigation may have established that the paper in question harbored research misconduct, or perhaps there was an honest error. Journals publish retraction notices and identify retracted papers in electronic databases, with reasons for retraction that are not always clearly stated. In case of honest errors, journals may retract and republish a paper or may publish a corrigendum.
- **Corrigendum:** The publication of a correction notice concerning a paper's version of record. A corrigendum refers to the correction of authors' error(s) in the research work where some elements of the paper may be affected, but its research integrity and main findings remain intact. A corrigendum requires approval by all authors and may be subject to editorial and peer review assessment.
- **Erratum:** The publication of a correction notice concerning a paper's version of record. The term erratum refers to the correction of a journal's error in the publishing process. A minor publishing error may be corrected by the journal without any author input, but authors should be notified.

The figure shows a tsunami of retractions (black vertical bars), with corrigenda (light gray bars) and expressions of concern (dark gray bars) showing large and small waves, respectively.
Source of data: PubMed search, November 2025. The citation counts are approximate, depending on the accuracy of coding of the terms searched.
PubMed is a freely available interface of the general biomedical research database Medline, which contains citations from around 5200 biomedical journals (ncbi.nlm.nih.gov/PubMed).

Health research is conducted in institutions such as universities, their affiliated hospitals, and laboratories. Journals are responsible for evaluating manuscripts of scientific writing before accepting submitted work for publication and for producing a version of record. They are also responsible for correcting the version of record, issuing expressions of concern while allegations of research misconduct are being investigated, and then issuing an exoneration statement, corrigendum, or retraction (with or without republication). Corrigenda have also increased in number in recent years (Box 1.1). Traditional publication practices keep journal evaluations secret, both before and after publication of the version of record. Retraction notices tend to be opaque, leaving unclear what occurred and what could have been done better. A complete overhaul of journal editorial and peer review systems is required to make them compliant with transparency and openness principles.

Institution: A clinical academic organization, e.g., a university or a hospital, where research takes place. Institutions have primary responsibility for the ethical and professional conduct of their studies.

Journal: An establishment composed of editors and other publishing staff who organize the peer review of manuscripts and their publication.

The research integrity focus of this book

Restoring trust in science is the greatest challenge in health research. Trust in science is taking a nosedive as there are daily notices and news about research misconduct and fraud.

Corrigendum: A correction notice concerning a paper's version of record when the error(s) in the research work do not impact the main findings.

Substandard, unethical, and unprofessional behaviors among health, biomedical, and life sciences researchers, reflected in the rising number of articles retracted, have implications directly for the clinical care of patients and public health policies. Something harmful may be introduced into practice, or something useful may be withheld due to the untrustworthy research findings reported in the literature. Evidence-based medicine, the pursuit of getting the best available research into practice, can only work if the evidence it deploys is trustworthy with respect to its integrity. Untrustworthy evidence leads to misguided practice.

Evidence-based medicine: The conscientious, explicit, and judicious use of current best research evidence in making healthcare decisions.

The COVID-19 pandemic triggered an unprecedented surge in research activity and output. It profoundly disrupted societies worldwide, causing millions of infections and deaths. Lockdowns and social distancing measures disrupted everyday life, shifted education to online platforms, lead to widespread student isolation, normalized remote working, transformed workplaces and urban patterns, and placed heavy financial strains on public funds through workforce furlough schemes in some nations. Mental health challenges escalated across all demographics due to uncertainty and prolonged confinement, while economies faced severe and broad-ranging difficulties.

While society was suffering restraints, scientists, backed by their institutions and funders, and journals were working extra hard to bring the pandemic under control. However, an extraordinary fact about their research efforts is often overlooked. In the race to beat COVID-19, they were competing against each other and were involved in publishing over 600 papers that were subsequently retracted (Retraction Watch, December 2025). Each of these cases of retraction represented a failure of the research integrity protection system that institutions, funders, publishers, and other organizations are supposed to have built in. The stakeholder organizations were competing for scientific glory. But they were also cutting corners in meeting their responsibility to maintain standards, prompting the emergence and spread of flawed research. The retracted papers tell the story of how the organizations all failed collectively to deliver their promise to society.

The above background led to the idea of this book. It consolidates specific guidance for inculcating a near–zero tolerance research integrity culture through an in-depth evaluation of case studies of research misconduct allegations.

Retraction Watch: A blog dedicated to reporting on research misconduct and tracking journal article retractions.

Research misconduct: Unethical or unprofessional behavior in research that is intentional, reckless, or negligent. Honest error is not misconduct.

Questionable research practices: Irresponsible research practices that are regarded as unethical or unprofessional but fall short of being defined as misconduct.

Raising research and publication integrity concerns

In this book, research integrity is defined as conducting and publishing research in line with established ethical and professional principles and standards. It acknowledges that lapses in integrity can stem from genuine mistakes rather than deliberate wrongdoing. Concerns may emerge at any stage of the research and publication lifecycle. Integrity issues can be raised by anyone, including whistleblowing by researchers, clinical staff, or study participants. Institutional audits and inspections, peer review (pre- or post-publication), sleuthing, online public commentary, independent academic or journalistic investigations, systematic reviewers, and others may raise queries (Box 1.2).

Whistleblowing plays a critical role in safeguarding research integrity and is legally protected in many jurisdictions. Complaints may be made anonymously and treated confidentially in line with organizational policies and procedures. Protection against retaliation is par-

Whistleblower: An individual, also known as the complainant, who reports a possible current or past breach of research and publication integrity for investigation.

Sleuthing: Investigation of possible research and publication misconduct and questionable practices by volunteer researchers.

ticularly important for junior researchers whose careers may be affected by the power exercised by those seniors against whose research practice they might have a complaint. To be eligible for this protection, complaints must be made in good faith and supported by evidence or reasonable suspicion. Malicious complaints may attract sanctions, whereas mistaken complaints made in good faith should not. Journals may undertake their own investigations, assisted by their publisher's research integrity team, or they may refer complaints to institutions, and funders and other bodies may also become involved in investigations. Sometimes, triggered by publicity in the news or on social media, organizations may initiate investigations without complaints being submitted to them formally.

Box 1.2 How concerns about irresponsible research and publication come to light

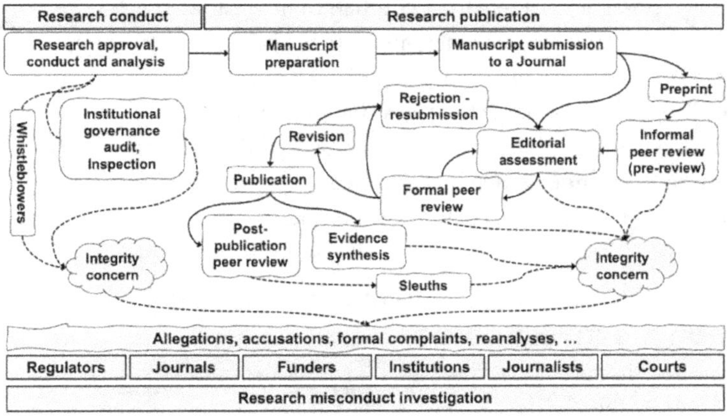

Figure: Solid lines: usual research and publication process. Dashed lines: integrity concerns and complaints.
See Box 1.3 for an outline of research misconduct investigations.
See Box 1.4 for a classification of irresponsible research conduct and publication.
Adapted from: DOI: 10.1201/9781003461401

All complaints made formally, or comments made publicly by sleuths, undergo an initial screening to determine whether there is a case to answer through an investigation. Frivolous, malicious, very late, or opinion-based complaints should be dismissed at this stage. There are many systemic problems in the in-house research misconduct proceedings, as they are not truly independent. Sometimes, investigating institutions err on the cautious side, initiating investigations despite weak evidence, exposing innocent researchers to professional stress unnecessarily. On other occasions, to protect themselves against reputational risk, they

Policy: A guideline or set of rules.

Procedure: Step-by-step instructions for implementing a policy.

may err on the side of leniency, setting aside complaints when there are serious suspicions of integrity breaches. If a complaint is deemed meritorious, a formal investigation should be launched according to the organization's research misconduct policies and procedures (Box 1.3).

Research and publication misconduct investigations

Research misconduct investigations are essential for protecting research integrity and the scientific record. They adjudicate whether a concern raised is found, establishing a research integrity flaw. Additionally, they establish if there was an honest error, or deliberate, knowing, reckless, or negligent misconduct, or questionable practice in research or publication. Along with scientific record correction, the investigations may impose other sanctions (Box 1.3). The burden of responsibility is huge. Investigation committees should be competent, as independent as possible, and free from conflicts of interest, with access to competent external experts where necessary. This is often not the case, and even the experts involved tend to have no legal training, so they make all kinds of mistakes. On re-examination in courts, judges have reached conclusions different from those of organizational investigation committees. Independent or external bodies are often better placed to investigate allegations of serious misconduct objectively.

Respondent: The researcher whose research conduct is the subject of a complaint or is being investigated.

Conflict of interests: Potential or perceived compromise in the objectivity or judgment of anyone involved in research due to financial or personal (non-financial) interests. Failure of declaration is considered research misconduct.

Box 1.3 How allegations of irresponsible research and publication are investigated

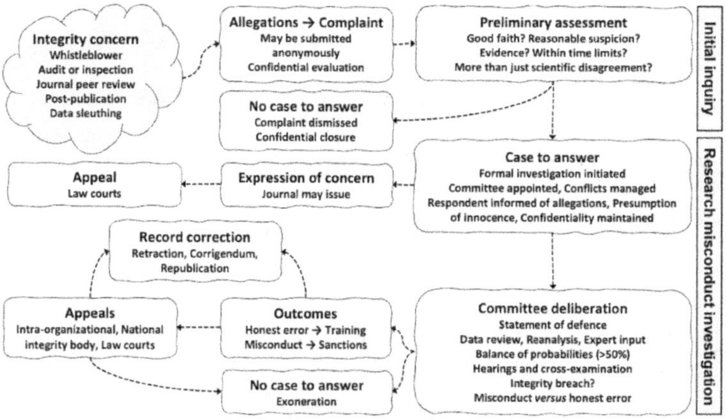

Definitions vary across jurisdictions. Note that honest error is not misconduct.
See Box 1.4 for the classification of research misconduct and questionable research practices.
See Chapter 3 for a case of misconduct in the investigation of allegations of research misconduct.
Examples of related flowcharts: DOIs: 10.24318/cope.2019.2.4; 10.24318/cope.2019.2.21.
Source: DOI: 10.1201/9781003461401

Both whistleblowers and respondent researchers have defined rights and responsibilities. Respondents are entitled to the presumption of innocence, disclosure of specific allegations, full access to the evidence, legal counsel, and protection against double jeopardy. Decisions are made on the balance of probabilities, not criminal or scientific standards of proof, raising the stakes for procedural fairness and transparency. Research and publication misconduct investigations are inherently high-risk. To be credible and just, they must make the distinction between honest error and misconduct. Strong governance, prevention through training and oversight, and harmonization of policies across stakeholder organizations are essential to maintaining trust in research. Investigation outcomes at one end of the scale may be complete exoneration or a finding of honest error requiring record correction and researcher retraining. At the other end, confirmed misconduct may be sanctioned with retraction, funding withdrawal, employment consequences, or referral to professional regulators. Sanctions should prioritize correction of the research record and prevention of future harm, rather than punishment alone.

The overwhelming majority of investigations into allegations of research and publication misconduct are conducted in strict confidence. As a result, they remain shielded from public view. Valuable opportunities to learn from these incidents and to repair the broken research integrity culture are missed if findings cannot be shared. In some circumstances, where organizations are forced to go public or if the law courts become involved, the details of research conduct and publication may be revealed. Sleuths, journalists, and independent researchers may also publish their investigations or reanalysis publicly. This book takes a look at some such cases (Box 1.4). It contains case studies concerning responsible research conduct and publication, drawing information from publicly available expert testimonies, investigation reports, legal judgments, and published papers. The chapters in this book cover a wide range of allegations of irresponsible research and publication practices, including both misconduct, such as serious ethical breaches, fabrication, falsification, and plagiarism, as well as questionable practices such as selective reporting, p-hacking, and spin (Box 1.5). The book explains how specific allegations of irresponsible research and publication practices have emerged and how they have been assessed, investigated, and resolved.

Balance of probabilities: Proving that something is more likely than not to have happened, i.e., over 50% probability.

Professional regulatory body: By law, health care professionals must be registered with a professional regulatory body to ensure they are fit and licensed to practice. Such bodies may undertake a fitness to practice investigation upon being alerted about a research integrity concern.

Selective outcome reporting: A difference in the outcomes in a published study compared to its ethics committee–approved protocol. Prospective registration encourages reporting of the result for the original primary outcome, even if it shows a statistically non-significant result on study completion.

Box 1.4 Book content and principal source information

Chapter number and title	Principal research integrity analysis sources
2. Metrics mania: Citation practices under spotlight in Salamanca	National independent investigation, journalistic investigation, published retraction notices, and internal institutional investigation
3. Research misconduct investigation: Conflict of interest and confidentiality breach in Utah	Court judgment
4. Responsible publication and research: Alleged editorial conflict of interest, and disputed data in Ohio	Court judgments, expert testimony presented in court, and published retraction notices
5. Post-publication clinical trial restoration: Lack of public editorial response in New England	Journal correspondence and independent reanalysis published in peer reviewed journals
6. Spinout roller coaster: Technology transfer in Washington	Court judgments and published retraction notices
7. All that glitters may not be gold: Image manipulation and resignation in Stanford	Independent investigation and published retraction notices
8. Alleged misconduct in charity-funded research: Breach of contract and an investigation in Portsmouth	Court judgment, published retraction notices, and publicly available companies house records
9. Authorial credit and accountability: Retraction and reported guest authorship in Amsterdam	Published retraction notices and reflective article by guest author
10. Institutional research culture: Alleged ethical failure and patient harm in Stockholm	External and internal institutional investigations, a repeat definitive independent investigation, court records, published retraction notices, and commentaries in peer reviewed journals
11. Copy-paste without citation: Allegations of plagiarism in a British journal	Published retraction notices and editorial by publisher
12. Professional regulatory investigation: Alleged ethical concerns and conflict non-disclosure in London	Professional regulatory investigation, journalistic investigation, and institutional inquiry

Sources are detailed within the timeline boxes in the chapters.
See Box 1.5 for the coverage of allegations of irresponsible research and publication conduct in the chapters.

Box 1.5 Coverage of allegations of irresponsible research conduct and publication in this book

Classification of allegations of research integrity concerns	Chapters
Misconduct	
• Ethical issues, including failing to obtain human research ethics committee approval, failing to obtain informed consent, misinforming participants to obtain their consent, and others.	**4, 10, 12**
• Fabrication and falsification.	**4, 6, 7, 8, 9, 10, 12**
• Plagiarism.	**11**
• Conflict of interest mismanagement by authors, editors, peer reviewers, ethics committee members, funding panel members, research misconduct investigation committee members, and research oversight committee members, amongst others involved in the research lifecycle.	**2, 3, 4, 5, 12**
• Breach of confidentiality.	**3**
• Unethical authorship, including guest authorship (naming someone who does not meet authorship criteria), ghost authorship (not naming someone who meets authorship criteria), failure of authorial accountability on expression of concern or retraction, etc.	**4, 9**
• Unethical publication practices, e.g., coercive citation practices, buying authorship through a paper mill, predatory publishing, etc.	**2**
• Publication process manipulation, e.g., editorial coercion, organizing fake peer reviews, sharing peer-reviewed information with others, coercive citation practices, conflict of interest mismanagement, etc.	**2, 4**
• Wrongdoing related to research misconduct investigation procedures, e.g., failure to undertake formal investigation or delay, etc.	**3, 4, 7, 12**
• Other serious deception or deviation, e.g., failure to disclose integrity concerns raised in research grant applications, giving false scientific information in company prospectus to investors, breach of research contract, misappropriating research funds and theft, etc.	**6, 8**
Questionable practices	
• Spin in the description of research findings, including displaying misleading figures of data, e.g., truncating the axes to give a particular impression, or overclaiming causation when interpreting findings.	**12**

• Selective reporting of outcomes and results including unjustified reconstruction of pre-specified outcome, failure to follow approved statistical analysis plan, and data analysis manipulations such as cherry picking, fishing expedition, p-hacking, etc.	**5**
• Self-plagiarism, including duplicate publication.	**11**
• Inadequate citation practices, e.g., unnecessary self-citation, inappropriate citations of works of others, etc.	**2**
• Authorship abuse, e.g., highly prolific authorship (without meeting authorship criteria), invented authorship (naming someone without their permission), failure to take responsibility after appearing as an author, etc.	**4, 9, 10**
• Other irresponsible research and publication practices, e.g., failure to engage in post-publication peer review, vague or incorrect errata, corrigenda or retraction notices, etc.	**4, 5, 7, 12**

Definitions and classifications vary across jurisdictions. Note that honest error is not misconduct. Some issues are covered in multiple chapters.
See Box 1.3 for an outline of research misconduct investigations.
See Box 1.4 for chapter list and principal source information concerning analysis of research integrity.
Sources: DOI: 10.1080/08989621.2014.958218. Classification adapted from: DOI: 10.1201/9781003461401.
The chapter listing per integrity concern is for indexing only; no allegation of research misconduct, dishonesty, or malice is implied or intended against any individuals, institutions, journals, or organizations involved in the case studies covered in the chapters.

The research ecosystem culture

Beneath the findings of individual investigations lies a more fundamental question: what kind of research culture allowed these research integrity breaches to occur in the first place? The lapses documented in the investigations are rarely isolated incidents; more often, they are symptoms of a deeper, systemic issue.

Health researchers are expected to uphold intellectual honesty, consistently acting ethically even without oversight. However, maintaining this standard across research planning, ethics approvals, execution, analysis, and reporting is challenging in environments where integrity is undervalued. Viewing adherence to ethical and professional standards as mandatory, rather than optional, is best reinforced through ongoing training programs. Promoting transparency and open science practices is key to embedding research integrity visibly. Valuable insights for enhancing research culture can emerge from well-conducted root cause analyses of allegations of misconduct and questionable practices in research and publication.

Research culture: The academic environment comprising the norms, values, expectations, attitudes, and behaviors within research organizations. Academic freedom, collegiality, collaboration, equality and diversity, research integrity, conflict management with openness, accountability and transparency are all features of the research culture.

Multiple stakeholders operate within the research ecosystem and share collective responsibility for safeguarding the research integrity culture. For all involved, individually and collectively, an article retraction due to research integrity breach represents a major failure. Simply blaming the researchers achieves little. Instead, the focus should be on drawing lessons to strengthen the overall research culture, which requires an element of openness rather than secrecy. Journals, institutions, funders, and other parties must improve communication and collaboration between organizations. Stakeholders must adopt a coordinated, rather than siloed, approach to prevent problems early. Cure is often impossible, as retracted articles are seldom republished, but prevention is feasible through sharing the lessons learned from root cause analyses. Institutions, funders, and journals should adopt aligned integrity policies covering areas such as human research ethics committee oversight, data and safety monitoring, analysis, and reporting, covering the full research lifecycle. This book attempts to generate answers to the questions about the concrete actions that organizations overseeing health research and publication should take.

Funder: Organizations such as government agencies, philanthropists, research charities, industry, etc. that provide funding for research under contract to an institution.

Societies: Non-profit organizations that seek to further a particular healthcare profession and the interests of their patients.

Education and training

Science is error-prone and influenced by human and organizational factors. Researcher education and training play a key role in constructing a research integrity culture that can deliver trustworthy evidence. Whether substandard practice is tolerated in the workplace can be easily determined by observing what the organizational environment permits. On being found out, individuals and organizations are often ready to issue apologies and promise a better future. However, mistakes keep repeating themselves. Zero tolerance turns out to be nothing other than an empty slogan in this situation. As organizations are required to keep misconduct investigations confidential, there is little they can learn and implement to avoid future research integrity flaws due to the lack of openness. How can research misconduct and questionable practices be prevented? Ideally, problems are best avoided either by preventing them from surfacing in the first place or by nipping the evil in the bud through establishing workable policies and procedures.

Examples of root cause analyses of real-world case studies of research and publication misconduct and questionable practices are few. This book fills this critical gap, providing a learning resource for improving responsible research conduct and publication, both for personal professional development and for formal courses delivered to large or small groups. The hidden curriculum is as important as or

Publisher: An organization whose business is to prepare and issue works, such as books, journals, etc., for public distribution. It has the responsibility to oversee ethical and professional publication conduct.

Open science: An umbrella term covering various initiatives like open access publications, open peer review, open research data, citizen science, etc. that encourage sharing, cooperation, and knowledge dissemination without restrictions.

perhaps even more important than the explicit curriculum outlined in the training courses provided. Learning from case studies is a powerful influence. Each chapter in this book builds on a case outlining ethical and professional principles and standards to guide research behavior and ensure compliance. This way, it builds a curriculum for teaching core virtues, including truthful intent, faithful adherence to duties, and avoidance of cheating. It covers how individual researchers, shaped by their personal morals and educational backgrounds, can navigate career pressures. Exercising intellectual honesty at every step in the research lifecycle is not an easy task. Open science, with its transparency toolkit including pre-registration, protocol publication, conflict of interest declaration, and data sharing, among other tools, makes honesty verifiable and explicit.

Transparency in research: Open research practices including prospective registration, adherence to study design, *a priori* statistical analysis plan, data sharing, timely and complete public reporting, conflict of interest disclosure, open research assessment, open publication practice, etc.

Chapter structure, sources, and AI disclosure statement

Each of the chapters outlined in Box 1.4 starts with a preamble to a case study concerning responsible research conduct. Inevitably, every case has many aspects of educational value. Each chapter focuses on a particular aspect and gives recommendations as key points at the end of each chapter. The sources of information are summarized in the case study timeline boxes. The information sources are publicly available. The chapters discuss the cases in the context of research integrity scholarship. The marginal boxes give brief definitions to improve understanding of the terms used in the text. The sources of the definitions are provided in the suggested reading. The glossary of terms with detailed explanations appears at the end of the book.

During the preparation of this book, generative AI tools, e.g., ChatGPT, Grok, Copilot, Gemini, Deepseek, etc., were used to assist with searching and summarizing literature. All outputs were reviewed and verified against primary sources to ensure accuracy.

Readership of this book

This book brings together, in a single resource, the key principles and standards of research integrity in the full lifecycle of health research. For experienced researchers, it offers a comprehensive overview of integrity considerations. The content is presented at an accessible level for those without deep expertise, primarily targeting health research students and practitioners, master's and doctoral candidates in health research, epidemiology, and statistics, as well as journal editors, peer reviewers, authors, university and hospital research administrators, and members of human research ethics committees (institutional review boards or IRB). Written in straightforward, non-technical language, the book is also valuable for a broader readership, including clinicians who enroll patients in clinical research, professionals from the pharmaceutical and medical device industries, patient and public involvement representatives, members of research oversight committees, research governance staff, systematic reviewers, guideline developers, funders of health research, medical and science journalists and bloggers, sleuths, and others engaged in the administration of health, biomedical, and life sciences research.

Chapter 1: Introduction – Key points

The following key points describe the overall purpose and structure of this book.

- Evidence is untrustworthy without research integrity.
- Evidence-based medicine fails to assess the effects of healthcare interventions without responsible research conduct and publication.
- This book describes the research integrity principles and standards with critical appraisal of real-world case studies covering the entire research lifecycle from conception to post-publication.
- Case studies in Chapters 2–12 are covered systematically, including structured tables describing the:
  - Timeline of research integrity concerns and outcomes with sources of evidence.
  - Actors and their research integrity roles.
- Key points organized by stakeholder groups at the end of each chapter include the following:
  - Specific advice for researchers about openness and enhanced transparency in research conduct and reporting.
  - Specific recommendations for journals and publishers to put responsible publication into practice.
  - Specific actions for the various stakeholder organizations to support a responsible research and publication culture for maximizing research integrity.

2 *Metrics mania*

Citation practices under spotlight in Salamanca

Research integrity: Undertaking research and publication following ethical and professional principles and standards. Responsible research and publication require compliance with regulations and avoidance of publication process manipulation. Integrity failures may result from honest errors or deliberate misconduct.

Research misconduct: Unethical or unprofessional behavior in research that is intentional, reckless, or negligent. Honest error is not misconduct.

Questionable research practices: Irresponsible research practices that are regarded as unethical or unprofessional but fall short of being defined as misconduct.

Citation: A reference to the original source of information written in an article.

Responsible research publication practices require accurate and complete citation of relevant references in the bibliography of scholarly articles. Citation counts are used to measure academic performance. At Spain's historic academic institution, the University of Salamanca, "systematic" and "deliberate" manipulation of citations was alleged to have taken place, according to an independent report commissioned by the National Research Ethics Committee of the Spanish Ministry of Science, Innovation, and Universities. An abnormal citation pattern had been noted first in 2022 in an independent research integrity blog, and following an alert by an anonymous whistleblower, a journalistic investigation took place. Subsequently, in 2024, a publisher's investigation led to the retraction of a large number of papers, 75 to be exact. The typically recorded reasons for retraction were "inappropriate or unusual citation behavior," "undisclosed competing interests," and "compromised editorial handling" in the retraction notices. There was no measurable change in the university's global academic ranking over the case study timeline. The *h*-index of the professor involved had reportedly increased from 33 to over 100 within the three years associated with the alleged citation manipulations. This chapter will cover alleged research integrity concerns related to coercive citation practices and publication process manipulation.

Responsible citation mandate

The recognized professional and technical standards governing citation and bibliography in scholarly publications serve as the foundation of the citation-based metrics used for academic assessment. As the research culture is highly competitive, researchers, institutions, journals, and funders are constantly vigilant about their performance and ranking. They also engage in citation practices that can boost their metrics. However, sometimes they go to the extreme, introducing irregularity in citation practices. Two common indices of academic performance that take citations into account are the h(Hirsh)-index and the impact factor. The latter's "official" version is known as the Journal Impact Factor or JIF for short.

The *h*-index is a powerful indicator. For a researcher, it is calculated by placing papers (co-)authored by them in rank order of citations (including self-citation in some databases), and the value *h* is

DOI: 10.1201/9781003655916-2

the number of the rank that is the same as the number of citations. So, an *h*-index of 33 means that the author has 33 published papers that have been cited 33 times or more. At the time of writing this book, some databases make no adjustments for article retraction in *h*-index calculation. The *h*-index grows as a researcher's career develops, and the numerical values have discipline- and subject-specific ranges. Hypothetically, disregarding discipline and subject for simplification and to create a basic initial understanding for non-expert readers, in a particular region where the *h*-index for early career researchers is 5–10, that for independent researchers at assistant professor and lecturer level could be 10–15, for established researchers at associate professor level it could be 15–30, for full professors it could be above 30, and for field leaders it could be above 60. Coercive citation practices may be deployed by authors, e.g., via unnecessary self-citation and influencing colleagues to cite them, to improve their *h*-index. The *h*-index varies depending on database characteristics, e.g., the value produced by the Scopus database tends to be intermediate between that obtained via Web of Science and Google Scholar. The *h*-index is not always documented in formal organizational policies and procedures as a performance metric, yet it has become a common currency for estimating academic prestige. It is deployed explicitly or implicitly by institutions in appointments, appraisals, and promotions of research staff, and by funders in research grant assessments and awards.

Impact factor is a popular statistic for ranking journals in order of perceived importance. It is calculated as the mean number of citations per article in a year, taking as a denominator the total number of citable articles published in the previous two years in a given journal. *Advances in Distributed Computing and Artificial Intelligence Journal* (*ADCAIJ*), an open-access peer-reviewed journal in computer sciences, had a 2023 impact factor of 1.6, i.e., the citable articles it published in 2021 and 2022 were cited on average 1.6 times in 2023 (including self-citation). The "official" Journal Impact Factor, or JIF, is produced by Web of Science, which is owned by Clarivate and is a global citation database of over 20,000 journals that meet its quality and integrity standards. Note that if a journal loses its spot in the Web of Science collection, it cannot have an "official" impact factor. CiteScore, another journal metric that covers a four-year time period, is produced by Scopus, which is owned by Elsevier and is another global abstract and citation database of over 25,000 journals selected by its advisory board. Journals in a field are divided into four equal groups or quartiles, Q1–Q4, based on citation performance using impact factor, CiteScore, or other citation metrics. Q1 (top 25%) is the top quartile, Q2 (25–50%) is above average, Q3 (50–75%) is below average, and

Institution: An academic organization, typically a university, where research takes place. It has the responsibility to oversee ethical and professional research conduct.

Journal: An establishment composed of editors and other publishing staff who organize peer review of research manuscripts and their publication.

Funder: Organizations such as government agencies, philanthropists, research charities, industry, etc. that provide funding for research under contract to an institution.

Google Scholar: A freely accessible web search engine that indexes scholarly literature across a wide range of formats and disciplines, aggregating nearly all major scholarly publishing.

Web of Science: A global citation database that includes journals that meet its quality and integrity standards. It issues the "official" impact factor to rank journals.

Q4 (bottom 25%) is the lowest ranking. Year-to-year changes should be cautiously interpreted. Journal editors may coerce authors into including references to their own journals during manuscript revisions to boost their own impact factor. Retracted articles are included in the denominator, but citations to retracted articles are excluded from the numerator. This means that retractions can lower the impact factor.

Every citation must be accurate, complete, and allow a reader to easily trace the original source. Citation is the mechanism by which proper attribution is made to the original source of an idea, text, or data. It protects intellectual property and prevents plagiarism. Citations should be directly relevant and substantively connected to the background, methods, and claims made in the published work. Citations included in the bibliography of any scholarly work must be free from pressure by supervisors, editors, or peer reviewers. The practice of exercising power to demand citations to one's work or journal as a condition of collaboration or publication is generally considered a form of research misconduct. Irresponsible citation practices, including inappropriate, irrelevant, misleading, missing, and inaccurate citations, make a mockery of a system that employs the above-mentioned indices. Over-citation to inflate metrics is a fundamental breach of integrity.

This chapter presents a case study involving allegations of irresponsible citation practices, combined with publication process manipulation and failures of conflict of interest declaration. The case highlights questions about institutional leadership and the responsibility of the stakeholder organizations in the research ecosystem to nurture a healthy research culture and provide oversight.

Scopus: A global abstract and citation database. It has a content selection and advisory board. It produces the CiteScore to rank journals.

Publish or perish: An academic culture in which institutions value the number of papers rather than their quality or their impact.

Inadequate citation practices: Erroneously included citations in published articles, including unnecessary self-citation as well as citations of works of others that are inappropriate, irrelevant, misleading, missing, inaccurate, etc.

A case study of allegations of citation manipulation

This case study summarizes information from publicly available reports of national, institutional, and journalistic investigations (Box 2.1) and discusses them in the context of research integrity scholarship.

The University of Salamanca, one of the world's oldest higher education institutions, founded eight centuries ago, celebrated for its history and stunning architecture, is regarded as a key pillar of Spanish academia. As a comprehensive research university, it stood at around 701–800 in the 2020 Shanghai Academic Ranking of World Universities. It hosted the Bioinformatics, Intelligent Systems and Educational Technology (BISITE) research group, and its associated *ADCAIJ*. The

Shanghai (ARWU) ranking: Academic Ranking of World Universities, one of the most influential global research-based university rankings.

BISITE research group lead was also the chief editor of the *ADCAIJ* published by the University of Salamanca.

Computer science and biomedical research have a powerful, dynamic, and synergistic collaboration that is actively contributing to progress in health care. A PubMed search covering a sample of all biomedical literature revealed over 50 papers by the BISITE research group in December 2025. Of the over 1000 papers of the BISITE research group lead listed in OpenAlex, ChatGPT estimated that up to 15% were related to biomedicine. The computer science–artificial intelligence field relies on conference proceedings and abstracts (summaries of oral or poster presentations at scientific conferences) far more than other research fields like biomedicine, which prioritize peer-reviewed long-form journal articles. Compared to journal articles, conference proceedings and abstracts tend to get fast-tracked in the publication process. They are extensively indexed in Google Scholar. In academia in general, the standard for research evaluation is the long-form article. However, in computer science, the short-form is a major publication channel.

In 2024, the BISITE research group lead was a candidate for the position of rector (president) of the University of Salamanca. He had fewer than 4000 citations with an *h*-index of 33 in 2016. In a three-year surge, from 2017 to 2020, the citations jumped from between 4000–5000 to over 30,000. Then, by 2024, the statistics had jumped again to more than 44,000 citations with an *h*-index reaching over 100 according to Google Scholar (Box 2.2). This represented a 300% rise. How did the candidate for the position of rector of the University of Salamanca get there? Was it the result of research productivity or citation manipulation? The Spanish National Research Ethics Committee, an advisory body to the Spanish Ministry of Science, Innovation and Universities, commissioned an independent expert report to get to the bottom of this puzzle. According to a Times Higher Education article covering this case, the title said it all: "Spanish rector 'created citation factory to boost reputation'" (Box 2.1).

The first public scrutiny of the citation record of the BISITE research group lead appeared more as a whisper than a formal complaint. In its March 2022 blog titled "How Critics Say a Computer Scientist in Spain Artificially Boosted His Google Scholar Metrics," Retraction Watch reported that around one in five of the BISITE research group lead's citations listed on Google Scholar were to his own papers. Google Scholar includes every indexed citation in the *h*-index calculation. Even if the author of the citing paper is the same as the author of the cited paper, Google Scholar counts it as a citation in its metrics calculation. Thus, excessive self-citation can artificially inflate the *h*-index.

PubMed: A freely available interface of the general biomedical research database Medline.

OpenAlex: An open-access bibliographic catalogue of research articles, authors, and institutions.

ChatGPT: Generative Pretrained Transformer, an AI-based tool that deploys on large language models.

Retraction Watch: A blog dedicated to reporting on research misconduct and tracking journal article retractions.

Sleuthing: Investigation of possible research and publication misconduct and questionable practices by volunteer researchers.

Whistleblower: An individual, also known as the complainant, who reports a possible current or past breach of research and publication integrity for investigation.

Box 2.1 Timeline of research integrity concerns: A case study of alleged citation manipulation in Salamanca

Dates	Brief overview of events
2017 onwards	**Alleged citation manipulation** *El País* investigation identified internal communications where the BISITE research group lead gave instructions to his team to include mandatory citations to his work and his journal *ADCAIJ* in their papers, establishing what it called the citation cartel. *Source: english.elpais.com/science-tech/2024-05-31/internal-messages-show-how-the-new-head-of-one-of-the-worlds-oldest-universities-organized-a-citation-cartel.html.*
Mar 2022	**First public expression of concern** Retraction Watch blog highlighted BISITE research group lead's unusually high numbers of self-citations in short conference abstracts, artificially boosting his *h*-index. *Source: retractionwatch.com/2022/03/25/how-critics-say-a-computer-scientist-in-spain-artificially-boosted-his-google-scholar-metrics.*
Apr 2023	**Whistleblower alert to *El País* and journalistic investigation** An anonymous whistleblower alerted *El País* about BISITE research group lead's practices. Its published initial findings a year later publicly raised concern about excessive self-citation. *Sources: english.elpais.com/science-tech/2024-03-20/the-aspiring-university-rector-who-wrote-a-four-paragraph-paper-and-cited-himself-100-times.html; ep00.epimg.net/infografias/2024/03/bisite-covid19/BISITE_Covid19-1.pdf.*
May 2024	**Independent official investigation** After BISITE research group lead announced his run for rector candidacy, the Spanish National Research Ethics Committee ordered a bibliometric expert report, which stated that there was "deliberate" coordination to artificially boost citations, according to the experts' analysis. *Source: digibug.ugr.es/bitstream/handle/10481/101049/Informe.v1.pdf.*

October 2024	**Retractions following publisher investigation** Springer Nature retracted 75 scientific papers of BISITE research group. It typically listed "compromised editorial handling," "inappropriate or unusual citation behavior," and "undisclosed competing interests" as the reasons for retractions in these cases. A related PubPeer comment stated that 98% of the references cited in one of the papers were authored by the BISITE research group lead or were papers published in *ADCAIJ*, the journal he edited. *Sources: DOI: 10.1126/science.zvmx7id. URLs: link.springer.com/chapter/10.1007/978-3-319-99608-0_66; pubpeer.com/publications/20F3EB39D0944D56FC42025D07A298; pubpeer.com/publications/1909393F3B0B9EB6690F5FCCD772D3.*
2025	**Post-retraction** The BISITE research group lead denied any wrongdoing, was appointed the University of Salamanca rector, and was in this post at the time of writing this book. The University's own investigation claimed that the levels of self-citation was within appropriate thresholds, according to its report. A separate report presented to its Governing Council claimed that the Spanish National Research Ethics Committee had overstepped its bounds. The Spanish National Research Ethics Committee concluded that this was a "missed opportunity to clarify the situation." The rector's Google Scholar profile was unavailable in 2025; the reason for its unavailability was not publicly documented (Box 2.2). *Sources: URLs: timeshighereducation.com/news/spanish-rector-created-citation-factory-boost-reputation; secretaria.usal.es/gesdoc/files/13487-P01_Informe_Comite_Expertos.pdf; secretaria.usal.es/gesdoc/files/13541-Informe_Rector.pdf; www.lagacetadesalamanca.es/salamanca/demoledor-informe-corchado-defender-honor-nombre-universidad-20240930141416-nt.html; www.ciencia.gob.es/dam/jcr:248d0a5f-ddc1-4d59-94a0-12c3df86cc4e/ComunicadoCEEI17Sept2024.pdf.*

See Box 2.4 for an outline of the research integrity roles of various actors in this case study and disclaimer. Sources listed above are a few of the many that have covered this case study. This box summarizes reported allegations and findings; no judgment is intended.

In March 2024, as he launched his campaign for the position of rector of the University of Salamanca, his citation record faced renewed scrutiny. An anonymous whistleblower who had originally informed the Spanish newspaper *El País* in April 2023 reapproached them in March 2024, providing the impetus for an extensive journalistic investigation. The first of the resulting newspaper articles was titled "The Aspiring University Rector Who Wrote a Four-Paragraph Paper and Cited Himself 100 Times." A short COVID-19 paper had inspired this title. The investigation claimed that the alleged irresponsible research conduct went far beyond simple self-citation.

In May 2024, the *El País* newspaper reported uncovering evidence of a calculated "citation cartel," including internal messages where the BISITE research group lead instructed his collaborators to systematically include references to his work in their publications. These demands required colleagues to include a high volume of references to his previously published work in their papers, reported the newspaper. Sometimes, according to *El País's* reporting, the demanded quotas explicitly required up to 20 citations to his papers per new publication. This quota was allegedly enforced regardless of whether the cited works were genuinely relevant to the new research. In July 2024, a post-publication comment on PubPeer, an online platform for post-publication peer review, noted that out of 49 total cited references in a paper by a member of the BISITE research group, 43 (88%) were found to be references to the BISITE research group lead's own works, while another five citations were to papers published in the *ADCAIJ* journal, which the lead edited. In another PubPeer comment concerning physical activity for the elderly, authored by members of the BISITE research group, 43 out of 52 (83%) of the cited references were to the works of the BISITE research group lead. The PubPeer comments stated that the conferences where these papers were presented were "organised and edited by members of the BISITE group, among other researchers." Furthermore, the *El País* investigation detailed the existence of seemingly fictitious academic profiles dedicated solely to compulsively citing his papers. By enforcing this systematic citation practice, the cartel allegedly created an artificial echo chamber where publications citing the lead figure increased rapidly, inflating the overall citation count close to the top position at the national level, according to the newspaper.

As the observation of the odd citation patterns transformed into a scandal, the national Research Ethics Committee of the Spanish Ministry of Science, Innovation and Universities took note. In May 2024, it appointed bibliometric experts for an independent investigation. The 131-page report, including 14 tables and 19 figures, also publicly

Power: Abuse of role asymmetry to influence junior colleagues to engage in irresponsible research and publication practices for personal gain.

Conflict of interest: Potential or perceived compromise in the objectivity or judgment of anyone involved in any aspect of research due to financial or personal (non-financial) interests. Failure to declare a conflict of interest is research misconduct.

Journalistic investigation: A systematic process of uncovering information on matters of public interest, such as research and publication integrity. It requires rigorous fact-checking usually involving multiple corroborating sources. Compared to general sleuthing, the work of journalists is governed by professional codes and regulations.

PubPeer: An online platform for post-publication peer review.

shared the data it analyzed. The report highlighted examples of disproportionate self-citation with numerous instances of short conference abstracts or papers containing dozens of self-citations. In some extreme cases, one- or two-page conference abstracts contained hundreds of self-citations. In some examples provided in the report, the exact same list of references appeared in unrelated papers. According to the bibliometric experts' report, the citation patterns were "systematic" and "deliberate" rather than the result of genuine scholarly necessity. They concluded in the report that the patterns were consistent with an attempt to inflate citation metrics and improve the academic curriculum vitae rather than scientific communication. As characterized in their report, these were "strategies based on questionable publishing conduct and bad editorial practices, if not on openly fraudulent practices" (translated from the Spanish document).

Retraction: Removing a published paper from the research record due, for example, to the discovery of a flaw in its integrity.

Box 2.2 Google Scholar *h*-index trajectory for the BISITE research group lead, showing rise and subsequent profile unavailability in the case study of alleged citation manipulation in Salamanca

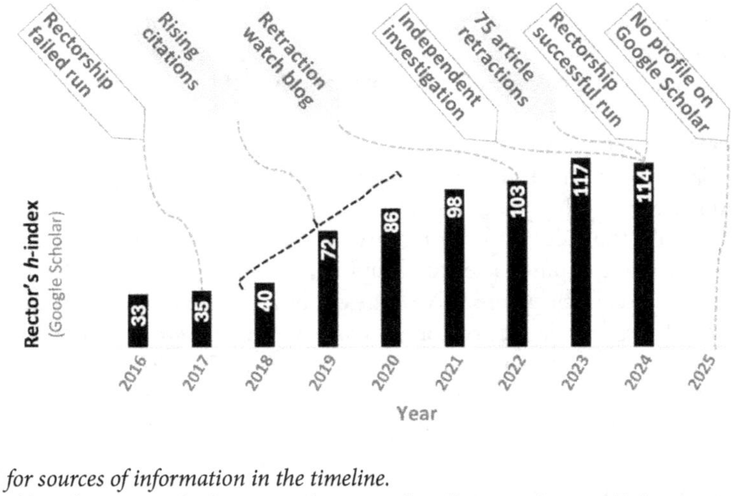

See Box 2.1 for sources of information in the timeline.
The historical h-index source: digibug.ugr.es/bitstream/handle/10481/101049/Informe.v1.pdf.
The reasons for the unavailability of the Google Scholar profile in 2025 were not publicly documented.

Box 2.3 Ripple effect in the case study of alleged citation manipulation in Salamanca.

Background

- Ripple effect is a situation in which an initial event triggers a series of consequences that affect increasingly distant parts of the ecosystem, just as dropping a stone into a pond creates circular waves that move away from the center, reaching areas not directly impacted in the first contact.
- Following article retraction, the ripple effect may trigger a cascade of consequences that extend beyond the retracted literature, e.g., contamination of evidence as the retracted studies continue to be cited, collateral damage to the "innocent" co-authors whose ability to obtain funding or enter new collaborations is potentially reduced, many retracted authors leave academic careers, institutions may suffer loss of funding or they may be fined, journals reputation may suffer or they may even close down after massive retractions, etc.

Initial case study event

- There were 75 article retractions following the publisher's investigation. The retracted articles had collectively cited the Salamanca rector over 1500 times, and his edited journal (*ADCAIJ*) over 500 times.

Institutional ripples

- The massive retraction pattern suggested a tight-knit set of recurring co-authors from the same circle, including students, postdocs, colleagues, and close collaborators in BISITE research group or its conference organizers in Salamanca.
- The careers or career prospects of many Salamanca co-authors would likely have been put at risk.
- The reputations of University of Salamanca and its BISITE research group were possibly put at risk (Box 2.4).

External ripples

- Outside Salamanca, the BISITE research group collaborators appearing in the retractions were possibly put at risk too.
- In one example, the vice rector for research of the University of Granada, Spain, a professor in the computer science discipline, co-authored with the Salamanca rector a retracted article where 50% of the citations where to the Salamanca rector's works. The Granada vice rector got named in the *El País* national newspaper article related to citation manipulation in Salamanca. Over 50 PubPeer comments addressed the Granada vice rector's co-authored work; these comments were discussed in a For Better Science blog covering the Salamanca citation manipulation allegations. There was no public record of engagement by the Granada vice rector in the retraction or the PubPeer comments.
- Observations concerning the Spanish National Research Ethics Committee and the publisher are given in Box 2.4.

See Box 2.1 for the timeline of the case study.

Sources: DOIs: 10.1007/s42001-024-00278-3; 10.1038/s41562-025-02154-0; 10.1126/science.caredit.a1500161; 10.1007/978-3-319-94649-8_43. URLs: forbetterscience.com/2024/10/25/schneider-shorts-25-10-2024-all-those-errors-occurred-inadvertently; pubpeer.com[search?q="vice rector's name"]; www.eldiario.es/castilla-y-leon/sociedad/editorial-nature-retira-75-articulos-rector-usal-no-confia-resultados-conclusiones_1_11738191.html; elpais.com/ciencia/2024-10-16/la-editorial-springer-nature-retira-75-estudios-del-rector-de-salamanca-y-sus-colaboradores-por-practicas-fraudulentas.html.

The publisher Springer Nature conducted its own investigation. Springer Nature is one of the world's leading academic publishers with a vast portfolio of over 3000 journals across science, technology, medicine, and other disciplines. It retracted 75 papers authored by the BISITE research group lead. Such a large-scale withdrawal of articles was interpreted in the investigation as indicating potential integrity issues across a sizable portion of the author's work. Some of the retraction notices listed "inappropriate or unusual citation behavior," "compromised editorial handling," and "undisclosed competing interests" as the reasons for retractions, according to the publisher's notes. The retractions serve to correct the scientific record by removing papers where concerns about the integrity of the publishing process were raised. The *h*-index of the research lead was reported to have increased from 33 to over 100 within a three-year period, according to Google Scholar (at the time of writing the book, the research lead's Google Scholar profile was not available; according to OpenAlex his *h*-index was around 75 in 2025 following the retractions).

Despite the events, according to public records, the lead researcher's campaign to be the rector of the University of Salamanca was successful in 2024, with no publicly reported institutional or legal sanctions at the time of writing this book. The ripple effect of the allegations and retractions was likely to have implications within his publication networks, both internally within Salamanca and externally (Box 2.3). At the time of writing this book, the *ADCAIJ* editorial board web page named him as one of the chief editors, but the publisher's journal home page did not, which could suggest a possible change in his role (adcaij.usal.es). His journal's impact factor was 1.6 in 2023, ranked in the Q3 quartile in the computer science–artificial intelligence field, whereas in 2020 it ranked in the Q4 quartile (Box 2.4). The University may have experienced some reputational damage, but its ranking, which stood at around 701–800 in the 2020 Shanghai Academic Ranking of World Universities, improved to 501–600 in 2025. Changes in institutional rankings, academic indices, or journal metrics are reported descriptively only; no causal relationship with the case study is asserted or implied.

For Better Science: A crowd-sourced project running a website on research integrity.

h(Hirsh)-index: A popular statistic to measure scientific output, taking account of citations, e.g., an *h*-index of 5 means that the author has 5 published papers that have been cited 5 times or more.

Impact factor: A journal statistic dividing the mean number of citations per article in a year by the total number of citable articles published in the previous two years.

Journal quartiles: A journal metric based on citation performance (e.g., impact factor, CiteScore, etc.) ranking all journals in a field into four equal groups, Q1–Q4.

Box 2.4 Snapshot: The reported dimensions of research integrity issues in the case study of alleged citation manipulation in Salamanca

Actors and their research integrity roles (described without assessing their adequacy or compliance with standards)	**Reported observations over case study timeline** (no causal inference implied)
Institution: University of Salamanca	
• Hosted the Bioinformatics, Intelligent Systems and Educational Technology (BISITE) research group, and its associated *Advances in Distributed Computing and Artificial Intelligence Journal* (*ADCAIJ*). • Responsible for oversight of the research conduct of its staff. • Responsible for investigating allegations of research misconduct under its published procedures. • Independent investigations looked into complaints that the professor leading the BISITE group (and *ADCAIJ* as chief editor) engaged in what was described as a "factory of publications and citations" involving his research team, allegedly enforcing a citation quota associated with disproportionate and irrelevant citations to his papers to artificially inflate citation metrics.	• Over 75 retracted papers. • Allegations of citation manipulation subjected to formal external investigations. • University's academic ranking improved. • The lead professor elected as the university rector in 2024. • The lead professor's Google Scholar profile was unavailable in 2025 (Box 2.2).
Journals and publishers: Springer Nature and others	
• Responsibility to oversee journals' publication practices, including citation practices and conflict of interest declarations. • The University of Salamanca published the *ADCAIJ*. • Springer undertook a publisher's investigation.	• Over 75 retracted papers. • *ADCAIJ* impact factor and quartile ranking unaffected.
Spanish National Research Ethics Committee	

• An advisory body to the Spanish Ministry of Science, Innovation and Universities, appointed bibliometric experts for an independent investigation into the alleged research misconduct. • It characterized the internal investigation by University of Salamanca as a "missed opportunity to clarify the situation."	• Produced an independent investigation report. • A possible loss of prestige as its findings were disputed by the University of Salamanca.
Whistleblowing, sleuthing and journalistic investigation	
• Retraction Watch noted the abnormal citation pattern. • An anonymous individual alerted the *El País* newspaper. • *El País* conducted its own independent journalistic investigation.	• Blogs and news stories published.

See Box 1.1 for research integrity terminology.
See Box 1.2 for how research integrity concerns might arise and Box 1.3 for an outline of a research misconduct investigation.
See Box 2.1 for sources of information and the timeline of the case study.
See Box 2.3 for the ripple effect of the allegations of citation manipulation.
Disclaimer: All factual statements are drawn from published literature and public records. No new allegation of research misconduct, dishonesty, or malice is intended or implied. The case study summarizes publicly available information and does not purport to determine liability or responsibility beyond what has been established in the cited records. References to individuals or organizations are made for academic discussion only and do not attribute intent or fault beyond the public record. When reporting changes in individual, institutional, organizational, and journal status or metrics, no causal inference is implied. The commentary and any opinions expressed are offered in good faith on matters of public interest concerning research integrity. Readers are encouraged to consult the original sources for full context.
University ranking data source: URL: www.shanghairanking.com/rankings/arwu/2025 (year).
Journal impact factor and ranking are based on Journal Citation Reports.

Research evaluation by citation metrics

Drawing from the public records cited above in this case study, the following analysis reflects on the implications for research integrity practice and culture. In the annals of academic integrity, few cases have sparked as much controversy as the one discussed in this chapter. Whispers of questionable practices outlined in a research integrity blog turned into a viral media story investigated by a national newspaper, an official national research ethics committee, and an international publisher. Even though no legal liability has been established, the case remains a cautionary tale, with ongoing calls for accountability and independence in investigations of research misconduct allegations. An outline of accountability as a research integrity principle is provided in Box 7.1. Drawing from publicly available reports, media coverage, and retractions in the case study presented in this chapter, what are the implications for the research integrity practice and culture?

The modern research environment is fiercely competitive. The quantifiable academic, driven by the pressure to gain a position in global rankings for themselves and for their institutions, may place undue importance on indices, scores, indicators, and metrics like the *h*-index and citation counts. While intended to quantify performance, the academic evaluation system creates strong incentives for organized manipulation of the citation-based evaluations. This case study discusses the official investigation report's finding of "systematic" manipulation of the bibliometric profile. Academic success should not be based on practices that could be seen as deception, such as alleged excessive self-citation, citation cartel organization, and publication process manipulation. When quantitative metrics become the end goal, they cease to be objective indicators of quality and become targets for maneuvering. The pressure for academic success should not be allowed to become associated with lapses in scholarship integrity.

Inappropriate uses of metric-based evaluations should be abandoned, according to several initiatives (Box 2.5). The Coalition for Advancing Research Assessment (CoARA) and Declaration on Research Assessment (DORA) both recognize the need for institutions and funders to improve the evaluations of researchers, eliminating reliance on metrics. Publishing and indexing systems, as well as institutional rankings, should have algorithms to proactively screen anomalous citation patterns, extreme self-citation, and high-density citation clusters that suggest organized cartels. The research integrity standards are critical for trust in science. Where there is suspicion, thorough independent investigations should take place. An example of independent investigation is presented in Chapter 7. Institutional leaders' conflicts of interest should be managed by removing them entirely from the stage so as to ensure that they are not in a position to influence or manipulate investigations into alleged research misconduct. Box 4.4 outlines the principles of conflict of interest identification and management. Chapter 10 presents a case study in which institutional bias is removed by investigating allegations at the national level. The case study in this chapter illustrates that metrics allegedly gained through manipulation may prove unsustainable and could be associated with reputational challenges and retractions.

Research culture: The academic environment comprising the norms, values, expectations, attitudes, and behaviors within research organizations. Academic freedom, collegiality, collaboration, equality and diversity, research integrity (ethics and professionalism), conflict management with openness, accountability, and transparency are all features of the research culture.

Accountability: A responsible research principle guiding individuals and organizations to be answerable for the research they engage in from idea to post-publication.

Transparency in research: Open research practices including prospective registration, adherence to study design, *a priori* statistical analysis plan, data sharing, timely and complete public reporting, conflict of interest disclosure, open research assessment, open publication practice, etc.

Box 2.5 Avoiding metrics mania: Some responsible research evaluation principles

Responsibility

- Recognize the negative effects of assessment with indicators as it may create incentives for gaming.
- Measure performance against the research missions of the institution, choosing indicators that target research group or researcher goals and context.
- Scrutinize indicators regularly and update them as with changing times once-useful metrics become obsolete.

Transparency

- Avoid black-box evaluations, keeping data collection and analytical processes open and simple.
- Allow those evaluated to verify data and analysis.
- Invest in the development and use of tools for identifying possible citation manipulation, e.g., c^2 or citation concentration index, RI^2 or the research integrity risk index that takes into account the share of self-citation.

Relevance

- Protect excellence in locally relevant research, avoiding language bias that can suppress the societal value assessment.
- Account for variation by field in publication and citation practices, normalizing indicators statistically.

Triangulation

- Quantitative evaluation should support qualitative assessment, not serve a substitute for informed judgment as indices vary by age, field, and database among other factors.
- Use multiple indicators for a more robust picture and avoid false precision.

Sources: DOIs: 10.1038/520429a; 10.12688/f1000research.140810.2; 10.1038/s41598-025-88709-7; 10.1007/s11192-025-05480-2. URLs: sfdora.org; coara.org.

Chapter 2: Metric mania: Citation practices under spotlight in Salamanca – Key points

Advice for researchers

- Prioritize genuine scientific contributions made with ethical and professional practices.
- Uphold the principle that citations must be relevant, accurate, and reflect scholarly contribution, not serve as a means of self-promotion.
- Avoid practices that artificially inflate bibliometric indicators like the *h*-index.
- Do not exploit power imbalance to unduly influence junior

colleagues. The responsibility for avoiding abuse lies with the powerful in asymmetric relationships (see Chapter 9 for power imbalances and authorship).
- Do not take part in citation cartels.
- Take responsibility as an author for the integrity of the reference lists.
- Declare conflicts of interest fully publicly (Box 4.4).

Recommendations for journals and publishers

- Ensure editorial and peer review process integrity.
- Implement robust checks to detect unusual citation behavior, high self-citation rates, and identical reference lists across disparate papers, particularly in conference proceedings.
- Whenever editorial process and peer review manipulation are suspected, launch immediate and thorough internal investigations for decisive response, such as mass retractions, to rapidly self-correct.
- Be vigilant about the identification and management of conflicts of interest (Box 4.4).
- Apply retractions as a neutral, corrective tool to maintain the trustworthiness of the scientific record.
- Exercise greater control over and give oversight to the editorial processing and peer review of affiliated conference proceedings.
- Invest in developing tools to detect citation manipulation.
- Scientific indexing services, e.g., Google Scholar and ResearchGate, should improve their algorithms and verification processes to quickly detect and filter out evidence of manipulation, such as the use of fake profiles or repetitive citation strings.

Roles of institutions and funders

- Reform evaluation systems urgently, moving away from reliance heavily or solely on the number of papers, raw citation counts, and bibliometric indicators.
- Disincentivize citation manipulation, shifting focus toward research integrity and societal utility.
- Invest in the development and use of indices for identifying citation manipulation, e.g., c^2 or citation concentration index (Box 2.4).
- Invest in the development and use of indices that make adjustments in institutional assessment for self-citation, e.g., RI^2 or the research integrity risk index (Box 2.4).
- Implement policies to support whistleblowing as a means of research culture improvement, allowing complainants to

come forward without fear of institutional or professional retaliation (Box 1.2).

- Implement independent investigations of allegations of irresponsible research and publication practices to avoid the biases associated with internal investigations (Box 1.3).
- Identify and manage conflicts of interest in internal investigations (Box 4.4).
- Cooperate with external investigations.
- Whenever organizational leadership is implicated in the outcomes of research misconduct investigations, the leaders themselves (see Chapter 7 for the Stanford University president's resignation) or their governance system (see Chapter 10 for the Karolinska Institute board replacement by the government) should take responsibility.

3 *Research misconduct investigation*

Conflict of interest and confidentiality breach in Utah

Research integrity: Undertaking research and publication following ethical and professional principles and standards. Responsible research and publication conduct requires compliance with organizational research integrity policies and procedures. Integrity failures may result from honest errors or deliberate misconduct.

When raising research integrity concerns within the workplace, confidentiality must balance individual privacy against the organizational need for a thorough investigation. At the University of Utah, a professor's allegations of research misconduct against a doctoral student were investigated and found to have insufficient evidence. However, according to court documents, the professor subsequently shared the allegations outside authorized channels, leading to a $160,000 libel verdict. Confidentiality helps to preserve the reputation of the parties involved in the investigation of the research misconduct allegations. The level of information sharing should happen strictly on a "need to know" basis. In 2013, the investigation of the professor's allegations against the research student had concluded that there was no case to answer. The institution, the University of Utah, had rigorously followed its research integrity policies and procedures. The professor, in his role as a whistleblower, was informed of the outcome with the instruction to maintain confidentiality. However, despite knowledge of the findings of the research integrity proceedings, the professor communicated his allegations to parties who did not have any legitimate reason to know. In 2015, there was a legal challenge to the poor handling of confidentiality. In 2024, the jury assessed that the failure to comply with institutional confidentiality protocols resulted in defamation. This chapter will examine a case study of how a professor came to be ordered to pay damages to his former research student whose information he shared beyond the appropriate professional channels after a research misconduct investigation.

Confidentiality: Keeping disclosed information private.

Confidentiality and research integrity

In the context of research integrity, confidentiality is a foundational principle. Protecting participant confidentiality is a key issue for all human clinical research. In research integrity policies, confidentiality is also incorporated in the whistleblowing and misconduct investigation procedures (Box 1.3). This approach is designed to protect both the complainant and the respondent from reputational harm.

DOI: 10.1201/9781003655916-3

For whistleblowers, particularly those at a relatively junior level, confidentiality is critical to prevent retaliation by the more powerful senior researchers against whom they might be complaining. This policy encourages the reporting of genuine concerns in good faith. Even when the imbalance of power and risk of retaliation is not an issue, the protection afforded by confidentiality is vital because unproven allegations can cause irreparable harm to a respondent researcher's professional standing, with consequences for financial status and career trajectory. Confidentiality is a nuanced matter. In this regard, it is important to recognize that making a statement (which turns out to be false) in good faith during the course of a duty, such as reporting suspected misconduct to the research integrity office, is not defamation. Such a statement should not be made with malice, i.e., with knowledge that it is false or with reckless disregard for whether it was true or not, and it should not be shared with those who do not need to know

Whistleblower: An individual, also known as the complainant, who reports a possible current or past breach of research integrity for investigation.

Institutional procedures for investigations of research misconduct allegations typically emphasize that knowledge regarding the identity of involved parties should be restricted on a "need to know" basis. When raising research integrity concerns within the workplace, the application of confidentiality involves balancing individual privacy versus the organizational need for a thorough, competent, objective, and fair investigation. Both complainant and respondent, as well as any witnesses, are expected to cooperate with an inquiry or investigation in good faith, maintaining the confidentiality of any records or evidence. Abuse of confidentiality would be the use or disclosure to others of the records or evidence that were shared with the expectation of confidentiality. A controlled breach of absolute confidentiality may be necessary when informing a respondent of the misconduct allegations made by a colleague complainant. This would be necessary to help permit the respondent to have the possibility of preparing an adequate defense. In this case, the information shared becomes privileged information that should be maintained in confidence perpetually. The outcomes of any research misconduct proceeding are similarly privileged, except when they need to be shared to take an action, such as the correction or retraction of an article.

Institution: A clinical academic organization, e.g., a university or a hospital, where research takes place. Institutions have primary responsibility for the ethical and professional conduct of their studies.

Policy: A guideline or set of rules.

Procedure: Step-by-step instructions for implementing a policy.

Respondent: The researcher whose research conduct is the subject of a complaint or is being investigated.

This chapter presents a case study of how a professor came to be ordered to pay damages to his former research student, whose information he shared beyond the appropriate professional channels after a research misconduct investigation.

Box 3.1 Timeline of research integrity concerns: A case of confidentiality breach concerning a research misconduct investigation in Utah

Dates	Brief overview of events
2008–11	**Doctoral studies** A student matriculated in the doctoral education program of the University of Utah and undertook research in the neuroscience department. In 2009, a grant (R43/R44 NS064661) was awarded to evaluate a device co-invented by the research supervisor. *Source: URL: reporter.nih.gov/search/rgVYd25sb0Sc8VP0VNQPiA/project-details/7745405.*
2012	**Supervisor's concerns** Supervisor privately expressed concerns about the student; their academic relationship soured after student's research findings did not support his hypothesis regarding the performance of a device which he had co-invented and in which he also had financial interest. According to court records, the supervisor had failed to make a timely declaration of interest. *Source: DOI: 10.3791/52554.*
2013	**Supervisor reported allegations of misconduct** The supervisor called the student "dishonest" and "untrustworthy" and barred her from his laboratory unless escorted according to court records. Later he formally reported "research misconduct" to the University's Research Integrity office.
2013	**Research misconduct investigation** The investigation during its initial deliberations determined that there was insufficient evidence for a formal investigation and instructed the supervisor to keep the matter confidential.
2013–14	**Confidentiality breach** According to court records, the supervisor ignored the confidentiality required and shared misconduct allegations with his daughter, professors at another university, and his own research staff.
2015	**Court case** Student filed a lawsuit claiming violation of her right to confidentiality and defamation.
2020	**Summary judgment** The court narrowed down the defamation case to the supervisor as an individual.

2024	**Court case conclusion: Student prevailed** Jury found supervisor liable for defamation and awarded the student $160,000 in damages. *Source: United States District Court, District of Utah Case number 2:15-CV-767-TS.* *URLs: storage.courtlistener.com/recap/gov.uscourts.utd.98282/gov.uscourts.utd.98282.237.0.pdf; cases.justia.com/federal/appellate-courts/ca10/20-4062/20-4062-2022-05-05.pdf.*

The description of events above pertains to the research integrity breaches, excluding other aspects of the case that are not related to these issues.
See Box 3.2 for an outline of the research integrity roles of various actors in this case study and disclaimer. Sources listed above are a few of the many that have covered this case study. This box summarizes reported allegations and findings; no judgment is intended.

A case study of breach of confidentiality

This case study summarizes information from publicly available court records, peer-reviewed publications, and the funder's repository of research awards, and discusses them in the context of research integrity scholarship.

The University of Utah is a public research university located in Salt Lake City in the western United States. In 2013, it ranked 85th in the Shanghai Academic Ranking of World Universities. It hosted the neurosurgery research group, where a doctoral student who had matriculated in 2008 became the subject of an inquiry into research misconduct allegations made by her supervisor in 2013. Her research involved the evaluation of a device that was co-invented by the supervisor, and together with the University's commercialization office, he also held an ownership interest in the company that manufactured it (Box 3.1). The supervisor had been awarded a prestigious innovation research grant to study the device. Regulations required him to manage the conflict of interest that arose, specifically to ensure that researchers did not feel pressured to produce positive findings in favor of the device. The student's research results did not align with the supervisor's hypothesis.

In 2013, the supervisor's relationship with the student deteriorated, and he barred her from his laboratory unless escorted. Later the same year, he formally reported a complaint about research misconduct to the University's research integrity office. The vice president for research integrity at the University was tasked, according to its research misconduct policies and procedures, with determining

Shanghai ranking: Academic Ranking of World Universities, one of the most influential global research-based university rankings.

Conflict of interest: Potential or perceived compromise in the objectivity or judgment of anyone involved in any aspect of research due to financial or personal (non-financial) interests. Failure of declaration is considered research misconduct.

whether enough evidence existed to open a formal investigation. The complaint lacked specificity, failing to provide concrete evidence to support allegations of research misconduct. Consequently, the research integrity office concluded there were insufficient grounds to initiate a formal investigation. The office explicitly instructed the supervisor to keep his concerns regarding the student's work confidential.

Despite the directive to observe confidentiality, the supervisor expressed his accusations to various parties who had no professional role in resolving the dispute with his student. He shared the research misconduct allegations with his daughter while she was a student at another university. He communicated these concerns to external colleagues at another university. He also discussed the allegations with members of his own laboratory. The court found that the act of sharing defamatory statements with individuals who did not have a need to know nor a legitimate professional interest in the matter was an abuse of confidentiality. Following the loss of her supervisor's support, the student was officially dismissed from the doctoral program in 2014, according to court records.

In 2015, the student filed a case in the law court claiming breach of confidentiality. The court documents signal that the supervisor did not provide a timely, formal, written notice of his financial conflict of interest. The records further indicate that the delayed disclosure formed part of the factual background considered by the jury when assessing his subsequent statements about the student's integrity. The student's research data failed to support the hypothesis that would have proven his device's value. The court considered both the supervisor's accusations that the student had been "dishonest" and had been "falsifying data" as well as the unfavorable research results. The jury's finding suggests that it agreed that the conflict of interest overrode the professional obligations, resulting in hostility.

Defamation: Discrediting someone or harming their reputation through a false communication.

In 2024, a jury found that the supervisor's actions constituted an abuse. The court records reflect escalating academic concerns and a breakdown in the supervisory relationship with the student. It was noted that he failed to verify the truthfulness of his accusations despite having full access to her laboratory data. The jury specifically found that the defamation was the result of willful misconduct, i.e., statements made regarding research misconduct were either known to be false or were made with reckless disregard for the truth. The verdict, totaling $160,000 in damages, reflected the defamation resulting from the breach of confidentiality.

In 2025, a year after the jury verdict had been covered in the media, the University of Utah's Academic Ranking of World Universities had dropped to 151–200 from 85th in 2013 (Box 3.2). Despite the court judgment, the supervisor's professional standing remained intact; he retained his university position and continued to remain active in funded research. His *h*-index was 90 at the time of writing this book, and his research continued to receive funding via national grants. Changes in institutional rankings or academic indices are reported descriptively only; no causal relationship with the case study is asserted or implied.

h(Hirsh)-index: A popular statistic to measure scientific output, taking account of citations, e.g., an *h*-index of 5 means that the author has 5 published papers that have been cited 5 times or more.

Box 3.2 Snapshot: The dimensions of research integrity issues in a case of alleged confidentiality breach concerning a research misconduct investigation in Utah

Actors and research integrity roles (described without assessing their adequacy or compliance with standards)	**Reported observations over case study timeline** (no causal inference implied)
Institution: University of Utah	
• Responsible for overseeing to research conduct of its staff and students. • Responsible for investigating allegations of research misconduct. Followed its research integrity policies and procedures when a research supervisor formally complained about a doctoral student. • Conflict of interest management.	• University's academic ranking dropped. • Supervisor ordered by court to pay $160,000 in damages for confidentiality breach in research misconduct investigation. • Supervisor remained in employment following the defamation court case and continued to receive research funding.
Funder: National Institutes of Health (NIH)	
• As the national health research funding agency, responsible for giving research integrity oversight to the awarded grants. • Conflict of interest management.	• Continued to award grants to the research supervisor at the University according to public sources at URL: reporter.nih.gov; no public record indicates that the funder took action regarding the defamation verdict (no inference is intended).

See Box 1.1 for research integrity terminology.
See Box 1.2 for how research integrity concerns might arise and Box 1.3 for an outline of a research misconduct investigation.
See Box 3.1 for sources of information and the timeline of the case study.
Disclaimer: All factual statements are drawn from published literature and public records. No new allegation of research misconduct, dishonesty, or malice is intended or implied. The case study summarizes publicly available information and does not purport to determine liability or responsibility beyond

what has been established in the cited records. References to individuals or organizations are made for academic discussion only and do not attribute intent or fault beyond the public record. When reporting changes in individual, institutional, and journal status or metrics, no causal inference is implied. The commentary and any opinions expressed are offered in good faith on matters of public interest concerning research integrity. Readers are encouraged to consult the original sources for full context.
University ranking data source: URL: www.shanghairanking.com/rankings/arwu/#### (year).
Journal impact factor and ranking are based on Journal Citation Reports.

Contribution of the funding effect

Funding effect: The pressure to prove a specific hypothesis linked to a secondary interest (financial or contractual) associated with funding.

Funder: Organizations such as government agencies, philanthropists, research charities, industry, etc. that provide funding for research under contract to an institution.

Drawing from the court records and jury verdict summarized above, the following analysis reflects on the factors that contributed to the confidentiality breach in this case study.

The need-to-know standards in investigations of research misconduct allegations in the workplace are well-known (Box 3.3). In this case, what factors caused the confidentiality breach? Why was there a continued dissemination of allegations after the integrity office concluded there was insufficient evidence for a formal investigation? The court records and jury verdict help shed light on this. The timeline indicates that the misconduct allegations emerged following research findings that did not support the performance of a device in which the supervisor held a financial interest. The case highlights how an unmanaged conflict of interest can potentially create the conditions for a breach of confidentiality and subsequent legal liability. There are established guidelines for the identification and management of conflicts of interest (Box 4.4).

Some whistleblowers may develop strong convictions regarding the validity of their allegations. They may also sometimes attempt to influence the integrity investigations and may even insist on accessing the records. The standard practice dictates that, beyond submitting their initial report, whistleblowers should play no further role in the inquiry process. In cases where the inquiry outcome favors respondents, disgruntled whistleblowers may turn to repeating their complaints formally in other forums. Following the internal complaint at the workplace, they may move on to journals and beyond. Going public is a confidentiality breach in misconduct investigations. When there is a conflict of interest, the complainant may lose objectivity and impartiality. A grant-winning professor whose student's research produces inconvenient results not aligned with what is hypothesized in the research grant awarded may resort to violating confidentiality over the integrity proceedings outcome. According to the jury verdict, publicly disseminating the accusations under these circumstances beyond authorized channels constituted defamation.

A breach of confidentiality in a research misconduct context is not merely an organizational policy violation; it is a legal risk that can lead to liability for defamation. There are many red flag indicators of conflict of interest observed in this case. The timing of the allegations was a potential indicator of the conflict of interest manifesting itself. The supervisor had co-invented and owned a stake in the company manufacturing the device that the student was assigned to research. The complaint had emerged after unfavorable research results, which had failed to validate the supervisor's device. Interestingly, the raw data had been available to the supervisor in the laboratory computer, but he never attempted to reanalyze it to confirm or refute the research findings made by the student before making formal allegations of misconduct. The jury's defamation verdict was based, in part, on evidence that the supervisor had characterized the student as "dishonest" and "untrustworthy" to third parties rather than examining the factual data recorded in the experiments. The student had been barred from the laboratory and told she required an escort. The student argued in legal filings that the requirement for a laboratory escort functioned as an isolation tactic that hindered her ability to conduct and defend her research. The research integrity office had concluded that there was no justification for a formal investigation and instructed the supervisor to avoid broadcasting his allegations.

Box 3.3 Need to know and investigation of research misconduct investigations in the workplace

Group	Need-to-know status	Explanation
Research integrity office	Full access	Oversight and management of the process
Investigation committee	Full access	Fact-finding and evaluation of evidence
Respondent	Partial access	Right to know allegations and respond to complaints
Whistleblower	Partial access	Right to know the outcome of the complaint made
General faculty and staff	No access	Risk of reputation damage and biased environment
External colleagues and family	No access	No role in the adjudicatory process

Procedures vary across jurisdictions.

Data sleuthing, post-publication investigation of possible research misconduct by volunteer researchers, works differently from workplace whistleblowing, as sleuths tend to be from external organizations and make their concerns known publicly.

See Box 1.2 for how research integrity concerns may arise and Box 1.3 for an outline of research misconduct investigations.

This case shows that the supervisor's subjective belief in the validity of the allegations does not constitute a justification for breaching a student's right to confidentiality of the final integrity inquiry resolution. The supervisor's professional obligation was to accept the finding of the investigation and maintain the confidentiality of the proceedings. The court records suggest a tension between the supervisor's financial interests in the device and the student's contradictory data, which preceded the breach of confidentiality. The background of the grant funding awarded to him and his commercial interest collided with the University's research integrity proceedings, which were not taking his side. He communicated his accusations to individuals who had no professional role in the investigation.

In the landscape of modern academia, the research translation from discovery to commercialization is encouraged. This approach is fraught with ethical complexities that require appropriate management. A financial conflict of interest creates a situation where a researcher's economic stake in a positive research outcome has the potential to compromise professional judgment. This background does not inherently constitute research misconduct. However, it can become a corrupting motivation. The key interpretation arising from this case is that unmanaged conflicts of interest may contribute to adversarial escalation in research integrity disputes. The reading of negative results no longer remains objective; these findings become an inconvenient burden that threatens commercial interests. This can create a dangerous feedback loop, leading a supervisor to make research misconduct allegations to discredit the student researcher. The research organizations, both institutions and funders, should have mechanisms in place for managing the risk to research integrity arising from this pressure to produce favorable results. Where there are failures to disclose conflicts of interest, there should be sanctions imposed.

Chapter 3: Research misconduct investigation: Conflict of interest and confidentiality breach in Utah – Key points

Advice for researchers

- Proactive management of conflicts of interest is a key responsibility. All colleagues involved in a research project should be informed of conflicts. ICMJE provides a form for disclosure of conflicts of interest. Independent research oversight by non-conflicted faculty offers a form of recusal (Box 4.4).

- Whistleblowing must take place in good faith. Allegations of research misconduct should be backed with evidence or reasonable suspicion. Without good faith, whistleblowers lose legal protection.
- The organizational research misconduct procedure is not a tool for the reconciliation of conflicts of interest.
- Adherence to confidentiality is a key standard in the research misconduct investigation process. Allegations should only be shared with individuals who have a legitimate professional role in resolving the dispute in the research integrity office (Box 3.3).

Recommendations for journals and publishers

- Promote strict adherence to conflict declaration and management standards such as those outlined by COPE, ICMJE, and WAME (Box 4.4).

Roles of institutions and funders

- Organizations must have a research integrity office and publicly available policies and procedures for research integrity, whistleblowing (Box 1.2), and conflict of interest management (Box 4.4).
- Allegations of research misconduct should be assessed rigorously, requiring specific evidence and supported by a sufficient rationale before initiating a full investigation (Box 1.3).
- The whistleblower should be asked to declare conflicts of interest.
- When red flags appear, organizations should pivot from a standard inquiry of a research misconduct allegation to a conflict management review.
- Any individual with a direct financial stake in the outcome of the research should be recused from the inquiry stage of misconduct proceedings. If allegations require data reanalysis, an independent third party should audit the raw dataset, bypassing the whistleblower (see Chapters 7, 10, and 12 for discussion on independent investigations).
- Funders should give clear guidelines for conflict management to awardees and monitor compliance.
- Funders should prioritize research integrity, reducing the pressure on awardees to produce positive findings.
- Organizations should impose sanctions on those who fail to declare conflicts of interest (Box 4.4).
- Organizations should impose sanctions on those who breach confidentiality in research misconduct investigations (Box 3.3).

COPE: Committee on Publication Ethics issues guidance to journals on responsible publication practices, including handling research misconduct allegations.

ICMJE: International Committee of Medical Journal Editors provides guidance to journals on publishing policies, such as public prospective registration, data sharing, conflict of interest declaration, authorship criteria, etc.

WAME: World Association of Medical Editors. It aims to improve editorial standards through self-regulation.

Transparency in research: Open research practices including prospective registration, adherence to study design, *a priori* statistical analysis plan, data sharing, timely and complete public reporting, conflict of interest disclosure, open research assessment, open publication practice, etc.

4 *Responsible publication and research*

Alleged editorial conflict of interest and disputed data in Ohio

Research integrity:
Undertaking research and publication following ethical and professional principles and standards. Responsible research and publication conduct pave the way for study methods and findings to be regarded as trustworthy. Integrity failures may result from honest errors or deliberate misconduct.

FFP:
Fabrication, falsification, and plagiarism.

Research misconduct:
Unethical or unprofessional behavior in research that is intentional, reckless, or negligent. Honest error is not misconduct.

Questionable research practices:
Irresponsible research practices that are regarded as unethical or unprofessional but fall short of being considered misconduct.

Fabrication – making up data and results – is one of the three cardinal research integrity sins enshrined in the classical research misconduct definition, abbreviated as FFP (fabrication, falsification, plagiarism). Inserting data unsupported by contemporaneous records into an article in response to editorial coercion mixes up irresponsible research conduct with irresponsible publication practice. A 2013 study published in a leading sports medicine journal reported injury dropout data that was later challenged in litigation, where human research ethics committee (Institutional Review Board or IRB) approval and informed consent also came under judicial scrutiny. The research misconduct and editorial irregularities became the subject of court cases that sought independent expert investigation. The expert report and litigation materials raised concerns that the journal's conflict of interest may have contributed to vulnerabilities in the editorial process. The journal retracted the disputed article in 2017 after issuing an erratum in 2015. The litigation resulted in monetary settlements involving a six-figure sum for the research site and a separate multimillion-dollar judgment against the journal's owner. Even after retraction, the paper in question has continued to be cited, something that perpetuated disputed information as noted in expert commentary. This chapter will examine a case study that illustrates how failures at multiple levels of the research publication ecosystem can allow unethical studies to get published, and disputed claims to creep in and persist in the body of the scientific literature.

Publish then perish

The term "publish or perish" refers to a competitive academic culture that recognizes researcher stature linked to publication output, both in speed and amount. Publishing scholarly papers gives visibility to scientists and their institutions. Academic employment and promotion measures publication numbers as a parameter capturing competence and productivity. Serving as an esteem indicator, it also plays a major role in academic status and rankings.

"Publish then perish" is another emerging related term. When publication becomes the reason for academic existence, those under

DOI: 10.1201/9781003655916-4

pressure to publish so as not to perish may be tempted to achieve their target via any means, including engagement in irresponsible research and publication practices. Then, if misconduct allegations are investigated and errors found, the publication may figuratively perish with its retraction. There were over 30,000 instances of retractions in 2021–2024 (Box 1.1). Thus, conformity with the "publish or perish" culture can contribute directly to the "publish then perish" outcome.

As the number of retractions has grown exponentially, the diversity of explanations for "publish then perish" has come to light. Many of these can be linked directly to the pressures of the "publish or perish" culture. The pressure originates from institutions that wish to demonstrate productivity to compete in university rankings, and this weight trickles down to academics. Prestige and reputation come from relying heavily on bibliometric indicators to quantify output, leading to a focus on volume over quality and gamification (Chapter 2). The desire for visibility and prominence can allow a parallel culture of cheating to creep in. This may include FFP, failure to meet ethical standards, authorship abuse, and other forms of misconduct and questionable practices (Box 1.5). Conducting human studies without human research ethics committee approval, failure to obtain proper participant consent, and reporting data characterized in an expert report as unsupported by contemporaneous records are the worst kinds of ethical and professional misconduct in research.

"Publish then perish" applies in the publishing business also. The standards of publishing, editorial, and peer review conduct are increasingly under scrutiny, with demands for transparency in the publication process. Many misconducts identified in retractions are related to manipulations in the journal assessment process, which tend to remain hidden due to its single blind nature, i.e., the identities of peer reviewers and sometimes even those of the editors are not revealed to the authors or the public. The very large number of retractions has forced publishers to rethink. In some circumstances, whole journals have perished or disappeared from the scene entirely, or they have been removed from the listings by agencies such as Web of Science after large numbers of retractions resulting from failures in ethical and professional standards in the publication process (Box 4.1). A related development is the investment by publishers in research integrity offices of their own. This signals the willingness of journals to investigate allegations of publication misconduct against themselves, as well as investigate allegations of research misconduct against authors, where institutional integrity policies and procedures are considered weak.

Retraction: Removing a published paper from the research record due, for example, to the discovery of a flaw in its integrity.

Institution: An academic organization, typically a university, where research takes place. It has the responsibility to oversee ethical and professional research conduct.

Shanghai ranking: Academic Ranking of World Universities, one of the most influential global research-based university rankings.

Impact factor: A journal statistic dividing the mean number of citations per article in a year by the total number of citable articles published in the previous two years.

Web of Science: A global citation database that includes journals that meet its quality and integrity standards. It issues the "official" impact factor to rank journals.

Box 4.1 Some journals perished following retractions: "Publish to perish" in the publishing ecosystem

***Tumor Biology* delisted from Web of Science**

- *Tumor Biology* is a journal of the International Society of Oncology and Biomarkers.
- In the years pre-2017 the journal was listed on Web of Science with an impact factor of around 3 and quartile ranking Q2 amongst oncology journals.
- In 2017 it retracted over 100 articles.
- The reported reason for the retractions was publication process manipulation.
- Its publisher was Spinger, but then it moved to Sage.
- At the time of writing this book, the journal remains delisted from Web of Science, but it appears in Scopus (note that a journal not listed in Web of Science cannot have an "official" journal impact factor).

Wiley discontinued four journals

- Wiley is one of the world's largest academic publishing houses, with over 1500 journals.
- In 2021, Wiley purchased the publisher Hindawi.
- In 2023, there were over 8000 retractions from Hindawi journals.
- The reported reason for retractions was manipulation of the publication and peer-review process.
- The Hindawi brand was discontinued.
- Four Hindawi journals with the highest retraction numbers were closed; the rest were folded back into the Wiley brand and of these some more journals were later closed.

See Chapter 2 for details of the "official" journal impact factor issued by Web of Science.
Sources: DOIs: 10.1126/science.aal1210; 10.1007/s13277-017-5487-6; 10.1038/d41586-023-03974-8; 10.1177/1010428317748815; 10.2478/fco-2022-0001. URLs: journals.sagepub.com/overview-metric/TUB; newsroom.wiley.com/press-releases/press-release-details/2021/Wiley-Announces-the-Acquisition-of-Hindawi; retractionwatch.com/2024/03/14/up-to-one-in-seven-of-submissions-to-hundreds-of-wiley-journals-show-signs-of-paper-mill-activity.

Publication process manipulation at the journal level bypasses or corrupts the independent, unbiased assessment of the manuscripts submitted. This may happen through the activities of external parties who hack the submission systems or influence the process by other means, such as providing fake peer reviews. Detection and prevention require investment in pattern checking to identify and counteract external manipulation. Another level of manipulation in-house, e.g., by conflicted editors, is a matter internal to the journal and the publisher. In this regard, theme or special issues handled by guest editors are considered vulnerable, but standard issues produced by nor-

Scopus: A global abstract and citation database. It has a content selection and advisory board. It produces the CiteScore to rank journals.

mally appointed editors have no particular safeguards. Conflicts arise if editors have a divergence between their interests and their responsibilities in the publishing process. If they have personal relationships with authors or financial relationships with companies that submit papers to their journals, then failing to disclose their conflicts of interest is a form of misconduct. Many journals have policies for editor conflict management, but public disclosure is rare, which makes it difficult to assess bias. Even the perception of a conflict of interest can undermine trust in the editorial process, so publishers need to be transparent in conflict disclosures and management. This is important because editors are the gatekeepers of scientific publishing. When editors' conflicts remain undisclosed, it can compromise the trustworthiness of the research published.

This chapter presents a case study illustrating how failures at multiple levels of the research publication ecosystem can allow unethical studies to be published and disputed claims to creep into and persist in the scientific literature.

Peer review: Evaluation of a scientific manuscript by others working in the same field, invited by journal editors before acceptance for publication as a definitive article representing the version of record.

Conflict of interest: Potential or perceived compromise in the objectivity or judgment of anyone involved in any aspect of research due to financial or personal (non-financial) interests. Failure of declaration is considered research misconduct.

A case study of editorial influence and disputed data

This case study summarizes information from publicly available court records, including expert testimony presented in court, published retraction notices, commentaries in Retraction Watch blogs, and peer-reviewed publications, and discusses them in the context of research integrity scholarship.

In the United States, Ohio State University is a major public research university. It ranked 63rd in the Shanghai Academic Ranking of World Universities in 2011, the year in which its Health and Exercise Science researchers conducted a study on the effects of high-intensity training. A manuscript of the article describing the study methods and findings was submitted to the *Journal of Strength and Conditioning Research* (*JSCR*) in 2012. That year, the journal impact factor was around 2, and it ranked in the Q2 quartile in the sports science field. Following peer review, editorial assessment, and several manuscript revisions, the paper was published in 2013. What followed was litigation and extensive scrutiny (Box 4.2).

Journal quartiles: A journal metric based on citation performance (e.g., impact factor, CiteScore, etc.) ranking all journals in a field into four equal groups, Q1–Q4.

In 2014, a local CrossFit-affiliated gym in Columbus, Ohio, filed a lawsuit in the Ohio Court of Claims against the Ohio State University for defamation. The case stated that the study conducted by the university's Health and Exercise Science researchers at the gym had reported participant dropouts due to injury in its 2013 *JSCR* paper; the injury data was disputed by participant statements. The gym

Participants: Individuals, also known as subjects, who meet the eligibility criteria and provide informed consent to participate in a research study.

had served as the research site in 2011. It was alleged in court filings that the reported injury data were inaccurate and harmed the gym's reputation. The gym had collected written certificates from the study participants confirming that none had dropped out because of injury.

Box 4.2 Timeline of research integrity concerns: A case of allegations of unethical research and disputed data in Ohio

Dates	Brief overview of events
2011	**Study conducted** Participants enrolled at a licensed gym which served as the research site in a CrossFit-based training study conducted by Ohio State University researchers.
2012–13	**Manuscript submission, peer review, editorial coercion, and disputed data insertion** Manuscript submitted with statement about human research ethics committee (institutional review board or IRB) approval and participant consent that were later found unsupported in the retraction notice. According to the expert report, injury data inclusion was required by journal editors, and the disputed injury data were inserted in the revised manuscript. *Source: s3.amazonaws.com/crossfitpubliccontent/Morreim_Initial_Report.pdf.*
November 2013	**Article publication** The version of record included: "Of the 11 subjects who dropped out of the training program, 2 cited time concerns with the remaining 9 subjects (16% of total recruited subjects) citing overuse or injury ... All the subjects provided written informed consent, and all study methods and protocols were approved in advance by the Institutional Review Board at The Ohio State University." *Source: DOI: 10.1519/JSC.0b013e318289e59f.*
2014	**Two court cases filed independently of each other concerning disputed injury data** Case 1: Gym vs Ohio State University, claiming defamation. Participants provided certificates confirming absence of injury. Case 2: CrossFit vs NSCA, claiming that disputed injury data were spread to gain a competitive commercial advantage. *Sources: retractionwatch.com/2016/10/19/ohio-state-crossfit-gym-make-six-figure-settlement-over-corrected-papers-injury-claims; law.justia.com/cases/federal/district-courts/california/casdce/3:2014cv01191/442865/394.*

October 2015	**Erratum** Stated: "the reasons for participants not completing follow-up testing, as reported in the article, were provided to the authors by the club owner. The club owner has denied that he provided this information. After the article was published, 10 of the 11 participants who did not complete the study have provided their reasons for not finishing, with only 2 mentioning injury or health conditions that prevented them from completing follow-up testing. In light of this information, injury rate should not be considered a factor in this study. This change does not affect the overall conclusion of the article." The court expert report described this as a vague statement. *Source: DOI: 10.1519/JSC.0000000000001121.*
October 2016	**Court case 1 conclusion: Gym prevailed** Court ordered Ohio State University to pay $145,000 in financial settlement. *Source: retractionwatch.com/wp-content/uploads/2016/10/potterf-settlement.pdf.*
June 2017	**Retraction and senior researcher resignation** Reason for retraction: "The study was not conducted under an IRB approved protocol for that study, as was stated in the article. Because the study was performed without proper IRB approval, the article has been retracted." Following this, the senior researcher resigned. *Source: DOI: 10.1519/JSC.0000000000001990.*
2017	**Post-retraction** Two further retractions of the same researcher group *Sources: retractionwatch.com/2017/06/30/researcher-tangled-crossfit-loses-two-papers; digitalcommons.wku.edu/ijes/vol6/iss3/7; digitalcommons.wku.edu/ijes/vol7/iss2/4.*
April 2020	**Court case 2 conclusion: CrossFit prevailed** Court ordered NSCA to pay $3,997,868 in financial settlement. *Source: law.justia.com/cases/federal/district-courts/california/casdce/3:2014cv01191/442865/416.*

See Box 4.3 for an outline of the research integrity roles of various actors in this case study and disclaimer.

Sources listed above are a few of the many that have covered this case study. This box summarizes reported allegations and findings; no judgment is intended.

Later the same year, in December 2014, CrossFit Inc., a privately held fitness company in Santa Cruz, California, filed a lawsuit in the United States District Court for the Southern District of California against the National Strength and Conditioning Association (NSCA), the owner of *JSCR*, where the high-intensity training paper was peer reviewed and published. CrossFit licenses its trademarked high-intensity training brand to affiliated gyms worldwide and certifies trainers and organizes the annual CrossFit Games. NSCA is a nonprofit professional organization that provides certifications, such as certified personal trainer, and publishes position statements, organizes conferences, and disseminates research via *JSCR*. At the heart of CrossFit's complaint was the allegation that NSCA disseminated inaccurate injury data in a way that harmed its reputation and benefited competitors; the court considered these allegations in its judgment. This legal framing appeared to transform allegations of research and publication misconduct into a case of fraud with commercial intent.

Research governance: The system set up by institutions to oversee that the conduct of research under their auspices is in compliance with ethical and professional regulations.

The above background set the stage for expert testimony about responsible research conduct and publication, which became public via the court documents. This was a 93-page report and a 14-page supplement covering many aspects of the study, from its approvals to its post-publication stage. There had never been any human research ethics committee or IRB approval nor informed consent obtained, the expert report explained. CrossFit was not involved in the design, conduct, or publication of the study in question, which took place in a local, independently owned and operated gym licensed to use the CrossFit training in Columbus, Ohio. The participants were recruited in the local gym that served as the research site. Ohio State University had the responsibility for research governance to oversee the study for compliance with research standards. There was no evidence of direct NSCA involvement in the study design and conduct. It had no organizational link to the research team or the gym site. The NSCA's role was entirely through *JSCR*, its journal. For *JSCR* distribution and indexing, NSCA had partnered with Lippincott Williams & Wilkins publishers.

Human research ethics committee: Institutional Review Board (IRB), set up under national research regulatory laws and tasked principally with the responsibility of giving formal approval to a research proposal and monitoring the ethical conduct of the research approved.

Box 4.3 Snapshot: The dimensions of research integrity issues in a case of allegations of unethical research and disputed data in Ohio

Actors and their research integrity roles (described without assessing their adequacy or compliance with standards)	**Reported observations over case study timeline** (no causal inference implied)
Institution: Ohio State University	

• Had the responsibility to oversee to research conduct of its staff and students, and the supervision. • Hosted the Health and Exercise Science research group whose article made statements about human research ethics committee (institutional review board or IRB) approval and consent that were later found unsupported in the retraction notice, and the expert report also described injury data insertion under editorial influence during revisions whose accuracy was later disputed in litigation. • Responsible for study participants protection at the research site. • Responsible for investigating allegations of research misconduct under its published procedures.	• Article retracted. • $145,000 settlement to the research site. • University's academic ranking dropped. • Senior researcher resigned from employment. • First author dismissed from graduate education program. • Observations made in court documents about its staff and students. • Further retractions.
Journal: *Journal of Strength and Conditioning Research* (*JSCR*), owned by National Strength and Conditioning Association (NSCA) and published by Lippincott Williams & Wilkins	
• NSCA had the responsibility to oversee publication processes in *JSCR*. • *JSCR* had responsibility for editorial and peer-review processes, which the court expert report criticized for being weak on due-diligence measures. • Editorial insistence on adding injury data not originally presented, according to the expert report. • *JSCR* was responsible for timely investigation of post-publication integrity concerns raised. • CrossFit alleged in court that the NSCA used its journal article to portray CrossFit as having elevated injury risk for competitive reasons.	• Erratum and retraction. • In court documents, the expert report characterized the erratum as vague and the retraction as delayed. • Financial multimillion-dollar settlement to CrossFit. • Journal impact factor and quartile ranking improved. • Editor retained and appointed emeritus editor after retirement.
Sleuthing	
• Retraction Watch and others blogged on the story.	• Blogs and news stories published.

See Box 1.1 for research integrity terminology.
See Box 1.2 for how research integrity concerns might arise and Box 1.3 for an outline of a research misconduct investigation.
See Box 4.2 for sources of information and the timeline of the case study.
All factual statements are drawn from published literature and public records. No new allegation of research misconduct, dishonesty, or malice is intended or implied. The case study summarizes publicly available information and does not purport to determine liability or responsibility beyond what has been established in the cited records. References to individuals or organizations are made for academic discussion only and do not attribute intent or fault beyond the public record. When reporting changes in individual, institutional, organizational, and journal status or metrics, no causal inference is implied. The commentary and any opinions expressed are offered in good faith on matters of public interest concerning research integrity. Readers are encouraged to consult the original sources for full context.
University ranking data source: URL: www.shanghairanking.com/rankings/arwu/#### (year).
Journal impact factor and ranking are based on Journal Citation Reports.

The journal's editorial process and the researchers' conduct both came under heavy scrutiny in the expert report. The report and court filings describe editorial pressure to add injury data during revision; the added data were disputed according to the expert testimony. The expert report also noted that the journal's ownership by NSCA created a potential conflict of interest, which litigation materials argued may have influenced how CrossFit was portrayed. The *JSCR* chief editor was an employee of the Ohio State University and passed over the manuscript handling to another editor as an individual conflict-management step. According to the expert report and court filings, this initial recusal was ineffective as he became involved again when the peer reviewer reports came in. The retraction notice stated that the study was not conducted under a human research ethics committee approved protocol as claimed. The expert report noted that the journal could have required sight of the human research ethics committee approval letter at the time of submission. There was no participant consent either, according to the report. Although the participants signed a form, it was not a consent form for the study submitted to the journal; it was for a different study. There was no prospective registration of the study. The ICMJE mandate for study registration before the first participant is enrolled has been in place since 2005. *JSCR* was not under the ICMJE umbrella.

ICMJE: International Committee of Medical Journal Editors provides guidance to journals on publishing policies, such as public prospective registration, data sharing, conflict of interest declaration, etc.

The journal's processes with respect to handling peer review and authors' responses did not appear to be genuinely independent, according to the court filings and expert testimony, which also described editorial pressure on authors during revision to add injury data. The originally submitted manuscript had not mentioned any injuries, and these data were added in the final manuscript revision; the accuracy of these data was disputed in litigation. Peer review and editorial revision requests became a focal point of later scrutiny regarding how injury data were introduced. No injury data had ever been collected or recorded on case report forms. According to the authors' statements submitted to the court, the senior researcher, the last-named author, admitted to having a limited contribution and not directly supervising the first author, who was a graduate research student. When the controversy broke, he clarified in his statement that he had not overseen the data collection or analysis, and that his role was more peripheral, giving input in manuscript editing. Based on his own statements to the court, his role – limited to manuscript editing without oversight of data collection or analysis – would not meet the ICMJE authorship criteria, suggesting a pattern consistent with guest authorship (discussed in Chapter 9). Participants provided affidavits under oath that they had not been injured. Court filings and expert reports stated that the first author was dismissed from his graduate program following the emergence of the disputed data.

Following publication, CrossFit had written to NSCA seeking clarification in 2014. According to CrossFit's filings and the expert report, the journal did not promptly investigate or act on challenges to the reported injury data. During litigation, it first issued an erratum and then retracted the article's version of record. The expert report stated that the journal's handling of the concerns did not align with COPE's recommended procedures for investigating allegations of research misconduct. According to the expert report, the erratum only noted that some injury data had been incorrectly reported. It did not explain that the disputed injury numbers had been inserted during revisions responding to peer review and editorial feedback. A retraction would have been the correct response instead of an erratum in 2015, the expert report explained. The expert report also noted that the erratum and retraction were inconsistently indexed. Because these were hard to detect and vague, the article continued to be cited as evidence of CrossFit's injury risk, perpetuating misinformation, according to the expert.

CrossFit argued in litigation that the NSCA's publication of disputed injury data about study participants recruited from an independent affiliate gym portrayed CrossFit training as unsafe. The lawsuit raised concern that the NSCA had influenced the publication process at its journal *JSCR* to insert the disputed injury data into the 2013 article. CrossFit's lawsuit characterized the disputed publication as trade libel and defamation, alleging that it harmed its reputation. The claim further alleged that the NSCA's actions were motivated by commercial interest, as CrossFit's rapid growth threatened the NSCA's market position in fitness certification and training.

Guest authorship: Listing someone who has not made a substantial contribution as a co-author of an article. Synonyms include courtesy, gift, and honorary authorship.

Erratum: A correction notice concerning a paper's version of record. It refers to the correction of a journal's error in the publishing process and is issued by the journal without the need for authors' approval. A **corrigendum** is a correction notice that requires approval by the authors.

Version of record: The final published version of an article in its definitive form with copyediting and typesetting completed, metadata applied, and DOI (digital object identifier) allocated.

COPE: Committee on Publication Ethics issues guidance to journals on responsible publication practices, including handling research misconduct allegations.

The outcomes for the various actors in this case study were uneven (Box 4.3). Ohio State University paid a six-figure sum in damages to the research site, and NSCA paid a multimillion-dollar settlement. The gym was awarded $145,000, and CrossFit was awarded $3,997,868. The senior researcher resigned following the article retraction. Two more of the research group's articles were retracted. In the Shanghai Academic Ranking of World Universities, Ohio State University was consistently ranked in the top 101–150 band globally during the 2021–2023 period, falling below the 63rd rank it enjoyed a decade earlier. According to public records, the journal and its editors faced no formal consequences. The *JSCR* chief editor was made emeritus editor after his retirement, and an outstanding sports scientist award was named after him by the NSCA. Despite the retraction in 2017, the disputed injury information continued to propagate; the paper has been cited over 300 times from 2018 to 2025 by Google Scholar. The *JSCR* journal impact factor in 2022 was around 3, and it ranked in Q1 quartile in the sports science field, rising from around 2 and Q2 respectively a decade earlier. Changes in institutional rankings, article-level indices, or journal metrics are reported descriptively only; no causal relationship with the case study is asserted or implied.

Google Scholar: A freely accessible web search engine that indexes scholarly literature across a wide range of formats and disciplines, aggregating nearly all major scholarly publishing.

Conflict of interest management

Drawing from the court records, expert report, and litigation materials summarized above, the following analysis reflects on the conflict of interest issues at the heart of this case study.

This case study covers many aspects of research and vulnerabilities in editorial processes. Interestingly, this case reveals how misconduct in scientific research and publishing can spill beyond academia, becoming the subject of litigation in the law courts. The court documentation and the judgment provide plenty of food for thought. The case demonstrates that misconduct may not be confined to individual researchers as authors but may be enabled by editorial influence. Expert report and litigation materials raised concerns that conflict of interest management may have contributed to vulnerabilities in editorial processes, the inability to respond promptly to integrity-related inquiries with misconduct investigation, and the delays and vagueness in the erratum and the retraction notice. The order of multimillion-dollar damages reflects the gravity with which the court assessed this case with respect to how NSCA's interests diverged from its responsibilities as a journal owner.

Policy: A guideline or set of rules.

Procedure: Step-by-step instructions for implementing a policy.

The judgment encourages the publication community to examine the need for a systematic examination of the explanations for the outcome. The article retraction is a sign or a symptom, a visible outcome rather than an explanation of the underlying issues. The identification and management of conflicts of interest, a frequently overlooked issue, is likely to be at the heart of this case. NSCA competed with CrossFit commercially, and this was a potential conflict of interest. The expert report and litigation materials identified this conflict; these documents discussed how such conflicts may have influenced editorial decisions. NSCA owned the *JSCR*. The publication process became a subject of scrutiny, including editorial correspondence and revision requests, which were examined for the possibility of bias against the effects of CrossFit training. Court filings and expert testimony indicate that the first author added injury data during revision and that the provenance of those data was disputed in subsequent proceedings (there were other flaws in the study submitted, e.g., failure to obtain human research ethics committee approval, but these were not picked up in the journal's assessment). The study with erroneous injury data was challenged by CrossFit following publication, but no formal research misconduct investigations were undertaken by *JSCR*. Once litigation began, the journal issued a vague erratum, according to the expert report. Finally, a delayed retraction notice was issued. The chain of events ended with financial damages awarded, recognizing that expert reports and court findings associated the publication issues with a conflict of interest. CrossFit alleged that the publication process was influenced by commercial rivalry; the court ultimately found liability for defamation. Expert report and court findings suggested that NSCA's commercial interests may have contributed to vulnerabilities in editorial processes, including disputed data, weak erratum, and delayed retraction. How could this be prevented in the future? Box 4.4 provides principles for developing policies and procedures to identify and manage conflicts of interest.

Transparency in research: Open research practices including prospective registration, adherence to study design, *a priori* statistical analysis plan, data sharing, timely and complete public reporting, conflict of interest disclosure, open research assessment, open publication practice, etc.

Accountability: A responsible research principle guiding individuals and organizations to be answerable for the research they engage in from idea to post-publication.

This case study demonstrates how misconduct can originate from errors and omissions committed by both authors and editors. Once research gets published, it remains available in the public domain after retraction. Even though logic dictates that retracted articles should no longer be considered further, their findings persist in the literature through citations post-retraction. This case and its outcomes underscore the need for reforms in the research and publication process with respect to research ethics committee approval verification, consent documentation, public study pre-registration, research student supervision, data transparency, editorial accountability, peer review openness, timely investigation of any credible allegations of misconduct, and prompt and visible correction of the scientific record to prevent the propagation of misinformation. Other case studies of ethical failures are covered in Chapters 10 and 12. It is important to focus on avoiding problems from occurring in the first place. Seeking to have sight of documentary proof of research ethics committee approval and a copy of a blank consent form would have been a simple editorial intervention that could have stopped the publication process in its tracks, in this case, right when the paper was first submitted.

Box 4.4 Conflict of interest: Some principles for identification and management

General

- There should be policies and procedures for complete and consistent disclosure at organizational level.
- Conflict disclosures should be standardized, e.g., ICMJE form.
- When conflicts exist, transparent recusal should be implemented for conflict management.
- There should be ongoing training for organizational leaders, researchers, editors, reviewers, research ethics committee chairs and members, funding panel chairs and members, etc.
- Who must discloseInstitutions: Leaders, researchers, collaborators, research ethics committee chairs and members, citizen engagement representative, study oversight committee chairs and members, research governance staff, etc.
- Journals: Editors, peer reviewers, other publishing staff, etc.
- Funders: Leaders, staff, funding panel chairs and members, peer reviewers, etc.

What to disclose

- Financial: Payments, shares/stock/options, royalties, support, consultancies, honoraria, patents, royalties, etc. (this item does not relate to research funding for the work, which need to be declared separately)
- Non-financial: Board memberships, affiliations, relationships, employment, etc.
- Personal: Competitors, colleagues, family ties, enemies, religious and other beliefs, etc.

When

- Institutions: Authors should disclose across entire research lifecycle, before and after publication, with updates periodically and as circumstances change.
- Journals: Editors and peer reviewers should disclose before involvement in a manuscript assessment.
- Funders: Funding panels and peer reviewers should disclose before involvement in a grant application assessment.

Allegations of conflict non-disclosure

- Investigate in the same way as that for any other research integrity concern (Boxes 1.2 and 1.3). Investigations should be independent, managing conflict of interest of investigators in a way that avoid the risk of bias.
- Fact finding should establish whether there was non-disclosure and determine if it impacted on any assessments.
- In case of serious deliberate conflict non-disclosures:
  - Institutions: Sanctions may be applied including in extreme cases termination of employment.
  - Journals: Published papers may be retracted, or corrections may be issued.
  - Funders: Funders may apply sanctions to either awarded individuals or contracted institution or both. Grants awarded may be terminated with recovery of funds, debarment or even referral to legal authorities, e.g., dual funding for same work may fall under the category of embezzlement or criminal intent.

See Chapter 2 for a case study of conflict of interest management in the investigation of allegations of research misconduct.
See Chapter 3 for a case study of an allegation of conflict mismanagement by a funded research supervisor in an institution.
See Chapter 4 for a case study of an allegation of conflict mismanagement in a journal.
See Chapters 5 and 12 for case studies of an allegation of conflict non-disclosure by the authors.
Sources: DOIs: 10.1186/s41073-025-00164-0; 10.1071/HC10171; 10.7189/jogh.08.010101. URLs: icmje.org/disclosure-of-interest; wame.org/conflict-of-interest-in-peer-reviewed-medical-journals.

Chapter 4: Responsible publication and research: Alleged editorial conflict of interest and disputed data in Ohio – Key points

Advice for researchers

- Always seek ethics committee approval or exemption. Always seek ethical participant consent unless an exemption has been granted. Undertake training in research ethics and consent. For transparency, provide research ethics committee approval letters with dates and consent documentation with participant information sheets (see also Chapters 10 and 12 concerning alleged ethical failures).
- Never insert data that are not supported by contemporaneous records, even under editorial pressure. This way, any allegation of misconduct related to data fabrication will be avoided.
- Resist editorial coercion; report undue pressure to the integrity offices of the publishers or to self-regulatory bodies such as COPE.
- Post-publication, actively participate in the investigation of

allegations and promptly correct the scientific record if required.

Recommendations for journals and publishers

- Editorial influence must be transparent and non-directional to maintain independence and the integrity of peer review.
- Recusal replacement of a conflicted editor as an individual conflict-management step is insufficient without systemic safeguards against editorial process manipulation (Box 4.4).
- Correct the scientific record judiciously. When data accuracy is fundamentally compromised, publication ethics frameworks generally regard retraction as more appropriate than correction (Box 1.3).
- Strictly adhere to standards such as COPE, ICMJE, and WAME. Incorporate editor training in research integrity, along with audits and other checks to enforce standards.
- Publish peer review reports and responses to help deter manipulation.
- Seek documentary evidence of research ethics committee approval and participant consent, providing these as supplementary material with published papers (see also Chapters 10 and 12 concerning documentation of human research ethics committee approval as an integrity check).
- Undertake prompt investigations focusing on authors as well as editors. Weaknesses in editorial processes and peer review may exacerbate or obscure research integrity problems.
- Create misconduct escalation pathways, e.g., establish procedures for confidential communication with institutions.

Roles of institutions

- Inculcate a research integrity culture that naturally encourages adherence to ethical and professional principles and standards (see Chapter 10 for an institutional action plan).
- Institutions have a primary role in giving oversight to research.
- Compliance monitoring must ensure that ethics committee approvals and participant consents are verifiable.
- Faculty training and regular updates in research integrity are essential.
- Reward research integrity, not just output and citations (Box 2.5).
- There should be a publicly available research integrity policy, including a policy for conducting investigations (Box 1.3).
- Engage proactively with editors when faculty misconduct is alleged.

WAME: World Association of Medical Editors. It aims to improve editorial standards through self-regulation.

Open peer review: An umbrella term for the various options available to make peer review compatible with open science principles.

Research culture: The academic environment comprising the norms, values, expectations, attitudes, and behaviors within research organizations. Academic freedom, collegiality, collaboration, equality and diversity, research integrity (ethics and professionalism), conflict management with openness, accountability, and transparency are all features of the research culture.

- Independent court-ordered investigations can be more forensic in analysis than internal investigations. Seek external, legally competent investigations to ensure robust assessment and to avoid conflicts of interest inevitable in internal assessments (see Chapters 7, 10, and 12 for discussion on independent investigations).

5 *Post-publication clinical trial restoration*

Lack of public editorial response in New England

Research integrity: Undertaking research and publication following ethical and professional principles and standards. Responsible research and publication practices pave the way for science to be regarded as trustworthy. Integrity failures may result from honest errors or deliberate misconduct.

Clinical trials that stop early and report positive findings based on composite outcomes can present challenges for interpretation. A landmark industry-sponsored clinical trial, undertaken collaboratively by a biotechnology company and an academic research organization affiliated with Harvard University, became the subject of controversy after publication in the *New England Journal of Medicine* in 2017. Having stopped early, it reported that the intervention was effective in improving a composite outcome. Post-publication peer review prompted an independent reanalysis via a Restoring Invisible and Abandoned Trials (RIAT) grant. Using data submitted to drug regulatory authorities for the purpose of licensing, the restorative authors reported discrepancies in death outcome adjudications. In a public call to action, they reached out to the lead author of the published article to correct the record. There was no response. The journal that published the original article also did not give any public response when informed of the restoration, according to the RIAT restoration authors. The *BMJ Open* journal published the restored analysis in 2022, and at this time, the original study authors responded with a rebuttal. This chapter will highlight the contribution of independent initiatives engaged in restoring scientific integrity amid unresolved debates over transparency, data sharing, conflict of interest management, and accountability.

Randomized clinical trial: A study involving random allocation of eligible, consenting human participants to intervention groups and their follow-up to compare group outcomes.

Misreported clinical trials

Evidence-based medicine: The conscientious, explicit, and judicious use of current best research evidence in making healthcare decisions.

Each year, approximately 30,000 randomized clinical trials are published worldwide. Among all possible research designs, the randomized trial sits at the pinnacle of the evidence hierarchy, providing the most robust foundation for strong recommendations in clinical practice and health policy. These trials, following approval of the protocol by the human research ethics committee, involve randomly assigning consenting, eligible participants to either an intervention or a control group, and then following them up to measure outcomes. A pre-specified statistical comparison of the groups for differences in the primary outcome determines the main trial result. For new

DOI: 10.1201/9781003655916-5

medicines, such trials provide the evidence required for regulatory approval to obtain market access.

It is noteworthy that far more clinical trials are registered than ultimately published, and many published trials deviate from their originally approved protocols and statistical analysis plans. It is not uncommon that, due to unforeseen difficulties in the implementation of the trial protocol or due to emerging findings during the course of the trial, studies fail to follow or need to deviate from the planned course envisioned for them in the protocol initially approved. In these circumstances, early termination and other protocol modifications, steered by independent committees advising trialists, may be justified. Any modifications to the original trial protocol and statistical analysis plan must be formally documented contemporaneously and require reapproval by the human research ethics committee. These details are often provided as supplementary materials in published trials. For instance, outcome switching without reporting the formal reapproval of the change is regarded as a research integrity failure. Inconsistencies between registered protocols, approved analysis plans, and final results reported in published papers raise serious concerns. These discrepancies were so ubiquitous in the past that mandatory prospective registration was introduced in mid 2005 (DOI: 10.1201/9781003461401).

Since 2010, close to trials have been retracted (PubMed search in December 2025). Evidence-based medicine, which fundamentally depends on the integrity of clinical trials, cannot tolerate deviations from ethical and professional standards even if they do not amount to research misconduct as formally defined and applied in retractions (Box 1.4). In response to the background of failure to register trials, trial non-publication, frequent non-adherence to the pre-specified outcomes and analysis plans, and the resulting high level of research wastage, several good-faith international initiatives have begun. Prominent examples include the AllTrials campaign, which advocates for the registration and full reporting of all clinical trials, and Restoring Invisible and Abandoned Trials (RIAT), which enables independent researchers to correct misreported studies. Tackling the problems highlighted above is not straightforward. Through their activities and projects, AllTrials and RIAT strengthen evidence-based medicine by helping to ensure that the scientific record is both complete and trustworthy.

RIAT is an independent international scientific initiative launched to combat two widespread problems: invisible trials that are undertaken but never published and abandoned trials whose published results are possibly inaccurate, incomplete, or misleading, i.e., misreported.

Retraction: Removing a published paper from the research record due, for example, to the discovery of a flaw in its integrity.

AllTrials: A campaign for all past and present clinical trials to be registered and their methods and summary results reported (alltrials.net).

RIAT: An international effort forRestoring Invisible and Abandoned (unpublished and misreported) Trials (restoringtrials.org).

Conflict of interest: Potential or perceived compromise in the objectivity or judgment of anyone involved in any aspect of research due to financial or personal (non-financial) interests. Failure of declaration is considered research misconduct.

Regulator of medicines: A formal body set up for official approvals of drugs and devices, e.g., Food and Drug Administration (FDA), European Medicines Agency (EMA), etc.

Proposed in a 2013 landmark *BMJ* article (Box 5.1), RIAT provides a structured, transparent process for independent researchers, also known as restorative authors, to access raw data for reanalysis according to the originally approved clinical trial protocol and analysis plan. Before proceeding and publishing corrected results, the RIAT process requires a public call to action, urging original authors to fix issues first, involving the original journal as required. If ignored, restorative authors proceed and publish an auditable restoration.

Box 5.1 An outline of the protocol for restoring invisible and abandoned trials (RIAT) with an example of the interactions between original authors, restorative authors, and journal editors

Outline of restoration protocol	Example restoration
Obtain clinical study reports and related data Document trial visibility and abandonment via literature searches, contact with original trialists, evidence of misreporting, or other documentation including but not limited to inspection of trial protocol and registration documents.	• A 2012 clinical trial, published following peer review in *Arthroscopy*, the official journal of the Arthroscopy Association of North America published by Elsevier, was found to be discrepant with its ethics committee approved protocol with respect to the primary outcome by a RIAT team. • *Arthroscopy* had an impact factor of around 3 and it ranked in the Q1 quartile among orthopedics and sports medicine journals in 2012. • The trial had begun recruitment in early 2008, but there was no public trial registration, something that was made mandatory from mid 2005 onwards. • The reported primary analysis was different to that given approval by the human research ethics committee in the original protocol.

Issue a call to action publicly Offer original trialists an opportunity to formally report or correct their work. Failure of engagement establishes the need for third party restoration.	• In 2019, a call to action was formally issued publicly in the *BMJ*, with RIAT restoration justified on the basis that authors were unwilling to make changes to the 2012 version of record. • The RIAT team had noted that there was "no evidence of any significant amendment to the protocol" and that there was an "inadequate disclosure on conflicts of interest" – an important factor due to the relationship of the original authors with the biotechnology company whose product was evaluated in the trial. • In a 2020 exchange of letters between RIAT team and original authors published in the *Arthroscopy* journal, the Editors' Note stated that the "decision is to not retract the initial publication."
Prepare and submit restored trial for publication Pre-submission inquiry, manuscript submission providing all underlying data.	• The restoration was published following peer review in the journal *Trials* in 2023. The prespecified, but previously unreported, primary analysis showed a statistically non-significant p-value. • In 2025, *Arthroscopy* had an impact factor of around 5 and it ranked in the Q1 quartile among orthopedics and sports medicine journals.

Sources: DOIs: 10.1016/j.arthro.2012.05.011; 10.1136/bmj.f2865; 10.1016/j.arthro.2020.01.004; 10.1016/j.arthro.2020.01.003; 10.1186/s13063-022-07049-3. URLs: www.icmje.org/about-icmje/faqs/clinical-trials-registration; restoringtrials.org; pubpeer.com/publications/36F70BA2835BD31AD64FE4CB49B3EC.

This box summarizes reported allegations and findings; no judgment is intended. When reporting changes in journal metrics, no causal inference is implied.

This chapter, in addition to providing a brief exemplar case in Box 5.1, covers a case study of a RIAT trial restoration, examining post-publication engagement in an influential clinical trial, focusing on the observable responses and actions documented in the scientific and public record.

A case study of a clinical trial restoration

This case study involves no formal finding of research misconduct. The following account is based on information collated from publicly available journal correspondence, peer-reviewed publications including a published reanalysis, and regulatory documents, and discusses them in the context of research integrity scholarship.

In the United States, academic research organizations often partner with industry to undertake research. One such organization, an affiliate of Harvard Medical School, commenced a multicountry randomized clinical trial in 2013. At this time, Harvard University ranked first in the Shanghai Academic Ranking of World Universities. In this partnership structure, the industry sponsored the trial, and the lead author of the published trial was a university professor. The idea was to design and conduct an academically driven trial, analysis, and event adjudication underpinned by industry funding (Box 5.2). In this case, the industry partner was a world-leading biotechnology company. Their product needed drug regulatory approval, and the trial was undertaken to provide the evidence required. The trial results were published in a 2017 article in the *New England Journal of Medicine* (*NEJM*), a journal of the Massachusetts Medical Society, which is a regional nonprofit professional association for physicians. At the time of publication, the journal had an impact factor of 79, and it ranked first in Q1 quartile among the journals in the general and internal medicine category.

In clinical research, a trial sponsor is the organization that takes legal responsibility for the initiation and management of a trial. It could be a commercial company, government agency, or institution. The sponsor's core responsibilities cover the development of the clinical trial protocol and methodology, compliance with research and data integrity standards, and participant safety monitoring, among others. A sponsor may delegate tasks to others, but it cannot delegate responsibility. Sponsor and funder are not synonymous terms. Where a government agency funds a trial, the sponsor is usually the institution to which the research grant is awarded under contract. The lead researcher is usually an employee of the institution awarded the grant. In an academic-industry research consortium, the commercial company may fund and sponsor the trial. In this case study, the biotechnology company was the sponsor. The lead researcher was a university professor. Researchers, as university employees, have an obligation to follow their institutional research integrity policies and procedures even when the employer is not acting as a trial sponsor.

Institution: An academic organization, typically a university, where research takes place. It has the responsibility to oversee ethical and professional research conduct.

Shanghai ranking: Academic Ranking of World Universities, one of the most influential global research-based university rankings.

Impact factor: A journal statistic dividing the mean number of citations per article in a year by the total number of citable articles published in the previous two years.

Journal quartiles: A journal metric based on citation performance (e.g., impact factor, CiteScore, etc.) ranking all journals in a field into four equal groups, Q1–Q4.

Sponsor: Clinical research regulations require that a sponsor take legal responsibility to make proper arrangements to initiate and conduct studies.

Box 5.2 Timeline of research integrity concerns: A case study of restoration of a clinical trial published in the *New England Journal of Medicine*

Dates	Brief overview of events
2013–2015	**Study conducted** The trial pre-registered, and 27,564 participants enrolled across 1242 centers in 49 countries. Trial terminated early and analyzed using a primary composite outcome measure. *Source: clinicaltrials.gov/study/NCT01764633.*
2017	**Manuscript submission, peer review, and publication followed by correspondence** Article published showed benefit of intervention and post-publication correspondence discussed composite outcome heterogeneity. *Sources: DOIs: 10.1056/NEJMoa1615664; 10.1056/NEJMc1708587. URL: pubpeer.com/publications/61828207992EF360AEF89FCCFFE0F9.*
2018	**Drug regulator public access policy** The laws governing public access to documents (redacted for confidentiality and privacy) in possession of governmental agencies became effective at European Medicines Agency. RIAT requested clinical study reports. *Source: URL: ema.europa.eu/en/about-us/how-we-work/access-documents.*
2019	**RIAT communication with trial lead researcher** RIAT call to action was published and asked, on three occasions, the lead author to share data and correct the conflicts of interest section of the trial publication to include all potential conflicts of interest. The communication stated that according to "ProPublica website, the main author … received payments during 2014–2016 worth over 130,000 US $" directly related to consulting on the intervention trialed. The lead author did not respond. No formal determination regarding disclosure adequacy has been publicly reported. *Sources: URLs: bmj.com/content/346/bmj.f2865/rr-12; bmjopen.bmj.com/content/12/12/e060172.responses.*
2020	**RIAT restoration grant awarded and drug regulator publicly released documents** The RIAT project was awarded a competitive research grant for trial restoration. Health Canada publicly released the clinical study report. *Sources: URLs: restoringtrials.org/riat-studies/funded-projects; clinical-information.canada.ca/ci-rc/item/207038.*

2021–2022	**Restored trial** The trial details submitted to regulators included protocol with amendments, the outcome definitions and measurement, and the statistical analysis plan amongst others became available. It became possible to evaluate the causes of mortality not previously reported. After independent outcome re-adjudication, it was found that when the trial terminated early, there was a non-significantly higher risk of cardiovascular mortality associated with the intervention. Manuscript submitted and restored trial published. The trial restoration authors stated that they emailed the New England journal editors to "inquire whether they would be interested in learning about our RIAT project … and also willing to correct the original article. In addition to the above-mentioned email, we also sent a reminder … but never obtained any response." *Source: DOI: 10.1136/bmjopen-2021-060172.*
2023–2025	**Post-restoration** The lead author and the biotechnology company defended the original analysis. The regulatory update continued to be based on the original composite outcome data. Update on the trial registration site did not contain the restored analysis. The biotechnology company performance on the stock market remained strong. *Sources: URLs: bmjopen.bmj.com/content/12/12/e060172.responses; timi .org/bmjopenresponse; clinical-information.canada.ca/ci-rc/item/269049; www.macrotrends.net/stocks/charts/AMGN/amgen/market-cap.*

RIAT (Restoring Invisible and Abandoned Trials) restorations URL: restoringtrials.org/riat-studies. See Box 5.3 for an outline of the research integrity roles of various actors in this case study and disclaimer. Sources listed above are a few of the many that have covered this case study. This box summarizes reported allegations and findings; no judgment is intended.

The trial was a major study, with 27,564 participants enrolled across 1242 centers in 49 countries. The paper published in the *NEJM* included a supplementary file appending conflict of interest declarations. It reported a significant improvement in the primary composite outcome, and this finding contributed to the evidence submitted for drug regulatory approval. Early post-publication correspondence in the journal raised concerns about heterogeneity in outcomes. A comment on PubPeer, an online platform for post-publication peer review, stated: "By casting such a broad net, the investigators seem to be seeking evidence from any of the four elements in the so-called primary endpoint." An independent team of researchers noticed underreporting of financial conflict of interest, identified inconsistencies in the published data when compared with the clinical study report

Participants: Individuals, also known as subjects, who meet the eligibility criteria and give informed consent to take part in a study.

of the trial, and suspected misreporting. Following the RIAT framework, the team publicly issued a call to action in 2019. RIAT urged the original authors to correct the record. There was no response received despite repeated outreach.

The RIAT researchers had pursued drug regulatory authorities to obtain the full clinical study report. The European Medicines Agency (EMA), Health Canada, and the United States Federal Drug Administration (FDA) all function under transparency laws to allow public sharing of documentation in their possession. Thus, RIAT was able to obtain data not previously reported in the published article via Health Canada. The original trial had adjudicated all potential endpoint events, including 870 total deaths, by an independent clinical events committee of the academic research organizations. An independent RIAT readjudication committee reviewed redacted narratives, applying the same standardized definitions as the published trial. There were discrepancies. Cardiac deaths were numerically higher in the intervention group, not highlighted in the original publication. Offers to the *NEJM* to publish a RIAT correction went unanswered. The RIAT reanalysis, published following peer review in the *BMJ Open* in 2022, called for full restoration of the trial record and urged clinical caution. Now, as the trial restoration came into the public domain, the lead author of the original paper responded with a defense of the originally reported analysis. The two studies remain available without any of the parties with a research and publication integrity role, including the institution, sponsor, and journal, coming forward to settle the matter.

PubPeer: An online platform for post-publication peer review.

Outcome adjudication committee: Outcomes, including adverse events, are best adjudicated by independent experts blind to participants' group allocation who standardize outcome assessment against protocol-specified criteria, minimizing the risk of measurement bias.

Measurement bias: Systematic differences between groups in how outcomes are assessed in a study. Bias or systematic error invalidates the study findings.

Box 5.3 Snapshot: The dimensions of research integrity issues in a case study of restoration of a clinical trial published in the *New England Journal of Medicine*

Actors and their research integrity roles (described without assessing their adequacy or compliance with standards)	**Reported observations over case study timeline** (no causal inference implied)
Academic-industry research collaboration: Harvard University partnered with a biotechnology company	

• An academic research organization, affiliated with Harvard University, partnered with a biotechnology company in a randomized clinical trial. • The biotechnology company was the trial sponsor. • The trial's lead author was an employee of Harvard University. • The collaboration partners had responsibility for research integrity and engagement in post-publication peer review.	• Restored trial findings differed from the original article. • The lead author remained in lead role in the academic research organization. • University's academic ranking was unchanged. • The biotechnology company continues to reference the original article in its business activities. Its market capitalization has increased over the period; no causal relationship with the case study is asserted or implied.
Journals: *New England Journal of Medicine* published by the Massachusetts Medical Society and *BMJ Open* published by the BMJ Publishing Group	
• Both are peer-reviewed journals. • As the journal publishing the original article in question, the *New England* journal was among the parties with a potential role in post-publication engagement; however, no public response or corrective action was reported following the trial restoration.	• The *New England* journal impact factor and quartile ranking were unchanged. • *BMJ Open* journal impact factor dropped and quartile ranking increased.
Drug regulators: European Medicines Agency (EMA), Health Canada, the United stated Food and Drugs Administration (FDA), and others	
• Health Canada shared documents in its possession publicly. • EMA and FDA procedures could not permit full sharing promptly.	• Post-approval appear not to have updated their documentation with the restored trial (at the time of writing this book).

See Box 1.1 for research integrity terminology.
See Bx 1.2 for how research integrity concerns might arise and Box 1.3 for an outline of a research misconduct investigation.
See Box 5.2 for sources of information and the timeline of the case study.
Disclaimer: All factual statements are drawn from published literature and public records. No new allegation of research misconduct, dishonesty, or malice is intended or implied. The case study summarizes publicly available information and does not purport to determine liability or responsibility beyond what has been established in the cited records. References to individuals or organizations are made for academic discussion only and do not attribute intent or fault beyond the public record. When

reporting changes in individual, institutional, organizational, and journal status or metrics, no causal inference is implied. The commentary and any opinions expressed are offered in good faith on matters of public interest concerning research integrity. Readers are encouraged to consult the original sources for full context.
University ranking data source: URL: www.shanghairanking.com/rankings/arwu/#### (year).
Journal impact factor and ranking are based on Journal Citation Reports.

This case study exemplifies persistent challenges in industry-sponsored trial reporting, documentation of conflicts of interest, the critical role of regulatory transparency policies, the value of independent reanalysis in restoring scientific integrity, and the difficulties faced by external researchers in correcting influential publications in high-impact journals from high-ranking universities that work in collaboration with powerful industries. The biotechnology company's market capitalization was approximately $127 billion in 2017, $140 billion in 2022, and $179 billion in 2025. The lead author of the published trial remains employed at the institution and continues in his role at the affiliated academic research organization (Box 5.3). His 2025 *h*-index was 162, according to Google Scholar. The University maintained its rank as the top research institution worldwide. The recent *NEJM* journal impact factor was 78, and it ranked second in Q1 quartile among journals in the category of general and internal medicine, whereas it had ranked first in 2017. By contrast, *BMJ Open*, the journal that published the RIAT restoration, had a recent journal impact factor of around 2, and it also ranked in Q1 quartile in the general and internal medicine category, whereas in 2022, when it published the restoration article, it ranked in Q2 quartile with an impact factor of 3. Changes in institutional rankings, academic indices, journal metrics, or market capitalization are reported descriptively only; no causal relationship with the case study is asserted or implied.

Market capitalization: The value of a public company traded on the stock market, calculated by multiplying the total number of shares by the share price.

h(Hirsh)-index: A popular statistic to measure scientific output, taking account of citations, e.g., an *h*-index of 5 means that the author has 5 published papers that have been cited 5 times or more.

Google Scholar: A freely accessible web search engine that indexes scholarly literature across a wide range of formats and disciplines, aggregating nearly all major scholarly publishing.

Post-publication engagement: Roles and responsibilities

Drawing from the public record summarized above, the following analysis examines the roles and responsibilities of the various actors, including researchers, journals, sponsors, and regulators, in post-publication engagement.

This case study highlights several research integrity issues, which revolve around transparency and accountability related to potential difficulties in academic-industry partnerships. Accountability as a research integrity principle is outlined in Box 7.1. There are many players with a role. The sponsorship responsibility, as outlined earlier, was

Accountability: A responsible research principle guiding individuals and organizations to be answerable for the research they engage in from idea to post-publication.

taken by the industry partner in this case. The lead researcher, as a university employee, has the responsibility to abide by institutional research integrity policies. The journal, too, has its own responsibility for publication process integrity and post-publication engagement.

There is no allegation of outright research misconduct made or investigated. Early termination of a trial does not indicate an integrity issue, but it does potentially statistically underpower the assessment. Discrepancy in outcome adjudication does raise a research integrity issue. If there is a mismatch between the assessments made by two different adjudication teams, as evidenced by the RIAT reanalysis, it could cast doubt on the findings reported. There are two results available in the public domain. How should the matter be resolved? Who should take responsibility for addressing the post-publication issue? This raises a question about the importance of accountability. Rather than attributing fault to any single actor, it is important to note that the visibility of post-publication engagement as reflected in the public record may affect transparency, interpretation, and trust in the scientific literature. How should the drug regulators, guideline makers, and evidence synthesis community handle the original versus restored trial versions? There are implications for evidence grading when generating recommendations.

Drug and device regulators are responsible for continuously seeking reassurances about the risks and benefits of medicines after giving approval. For this, they usually seek evidence from post-authorization studies. Are restorations of trials originally evaluated for regulatory approval also an element of this evidence? Based on publicly available information, drug regulators do not appear to have publicly considered the academic debate arising from the RIAT trial restoration in their decision-making. Whenever they take an interest in it as part of post-approval follow-up, they would likely ask the industry sponsor to respond to the published RIAT trial restoration. Such communication will most probably be considered commercially sensitive and will fall within confidentiality protection. Regulatory processes may involve internal considerations not reflected in public documents.

In a situation where there is divergence of findings between the original and the restored trial, the institutions and the journals involved have a responsibility in terms of their accountability. From the perspective of research integrity scholarship, non-engagement with post-publication inquiries may be considered inconsistent with norms of scientific openness. In this regard, the original journal's non-response to the RIAT restoration is a notable finding (see Box 5.1 for an example of the interactions between original authors, restorative authors, and journal editors). However, journals may have internal

Transparency in research: Open research practices including prospective registration, adherence to study design, *a priori* statistical analysis plan, data sharing, timely and complete public reporting, conflict of interest disclosure, open research assessment, open publication practice, etc.

Expression of concern: A note published by a journal to inform readers of there being the possibility of a concern about the integrity of a paper.

Corrigendum: A correction notice concerning a paper's version of record when the error(s) in the research work do not impact the main findings.

processes for evaluating such inquiries that are not publicly visible. Public critiques have questioned whether the conflict of interest disclosures in the original publication fully reflected all relevant financial relationships, raising broader issues about disclosure completeness. In this case study, the specific roles of the sponsor, the institution, and the journal in conflict of interest management appear to be unclear. The awards given by commercial sponsors to researchers are usually channeled through institutions via contractual arrangements. Regardless of whether such contracts enjoy privileged status, the issue of accountability and conflict of interest management at the organizational level remains key to custodianship of research integrity. In some countries, laws require that, for transparency, manufacturers of drugs, devices, biologicals, or medical supplies report payments made for consulting fees, speaking honoraria, meals, travel, etc., to doctors. See Box 4.4 for some principles for conflict identification and management.

Erratum: A correction notice concerning a paper's version of record. It refers to the correction of a journal's error in the publishing process and is issued by the journal without the need for authors' approval.

What roles should journals play? To ensure ethical and professional publishing standards, there are advisory bodies for self-regulation, including the Committee on Publication Ethics (COPE), the International Committee of Medical Journal Editors (ICMJE), and the World Association of Medical Editors (WAME). They advise on both conflict of interest management and post-publication engagement. Their guidance offers recommendations for best practices, not strict mandates, and permits editorial discretion. Journals should play a role in seeking clarity from the parties involved when concerns about conflict of interest disclosure or data discrepancy are raised post-publication (Box 5.1). A browse of the original article page in the *NEJM* confirms no expressions of concern, corrigenda, or errata at the time of writing this book. The PubPeer comments also do not have any response from the journal. The discrepancies highlighted may be viewed by the *NEJM* as non-material, justifying inaction as they do not constitute proven misconduct. No formal editorial ethics violation complaint has ever been publicized against the journal. These inactions may be interpreted by some commentators as reflecting broader tensions between journal-institution prestige and the need for engagement in the post-publication correction processes.

COPE: Committee on Publication Ethics issues guidance to journals on responsible publication practices, including handling research misconduct allegations.

ICMJE: International Committee of Medical Journal Editors provides guidance to journals on publishing policies, such as public prospective registration, data sharing, conflict of interest declaration, etc.

The above discrepancy has been labeled as publication asymmetry (Box 5.4). This term describes the imbalance in scientific publishing where original research is readily accepted and amplified in high-prestige journals, while concerns, criticisms, reanalyses, or corrections face major barriers. Those raising concerns have to expend disproportionate time and resources with little guarantee of equivalent visibility or impact. This creates a bias favoring initial claims (whether flawed or not) over challenges. Authors, institutions, sponsors, and journals resist engagement in post-publication peer review in case the revisions required undermine the originally published work, perpetuating potential errors in the literature and possibly also in practice and policies. This case study illustrates a pattern in which original findings from prestigious organizations receive significant visibility, while subsequent efforts to investigate research integrity may face challenges in achieving equivalent recognition.

WAME: World Association of Medical Editors. It aims to improve editorial standards through self-regulation.

Box 5.4 Publication asymmetry: Original glory *versus* post-publication research integrity concern

Description

- Publication asymmetry refers to the imbalance in scientific publishing where original research is readily accepted and promoted in prestigious journals, while criticisms, replications, or corrections require disproportionate effort from critics and face barriers to equivalent visibility or publication.

Causes

- Journals incentivize novel, positive results over critiques; authors and editors resist changes to published work to avoid undermining prestige.
- Variability in editorial capacity, workload pressures, and priorities amongst journals impacts on the speed, transparency, and completion of post-publication engagement once concerns come to light.
- Asymmetry in effort (original work is resource-intensive, but criticism is quicker) may be linked to outcome (original work finds high-ranking journal, but criticism is hard to publish).

Consequence

- Distorted scientific literature where errors may persist.
- Misleading clinical practice; for example, clinicians may be misinformed by end-point mislabeling.
- Long delays before erroneous papers are corrected or retracted.

Solution

- Promote open data sharing, encourage journals to publish critiques more readily and engage in post-publication peer review, independent initiatives like RIAT to restore misreported trials, among other open science practices.

See Chapters 7, 10, and 12 for other examples of possible publication asymmetry.

Sources: DOIs: 10.1136/bmj.f2865; 10.1136/bmjebm-2018-110917. URL: statmodeling.stat.columbia.edu/2019/06/17/the-publication-asymmetry-what-happens-if-the-new-england-journal-of-medicine-publishes-something-that-you-think-is-wrong.

Chapter 5: Post-publication clinical trial restoration: Lack of public editorial response in New England – Key points

Advice for researchers

- Follow the approved study protocol to the letter, and where justifiable modifications are needed, document them contemporaneously, seeking reapproval as required.
- Prioritize transparent, independent, blinded event adjudication, reducing the risks of bias and post-publication inquiries.
- Be prepared to share data and the underpinning case report forms, appropriately redacted.
- Engage in addressing post-publication critiques, responding promptly to concerns raised or calls to action, as nonresponse erodes trust.
- Always disclose and manage conflicts of interest rigorously (Box 4.4). Even when disclosures are made, perceived biases arising from concerns about incomplete disclosure or from sponsor ties can fuel skepticism.
- Clinical researchers, as key opinion leaders, have a greater duty for complete and transparent disclosures. In some jurisdictions, such as the United States, the public can check payments received by doctors. Make enhanced disclosures, going over and above the minimum declaration requirements. Do not leave room for doubt.

Recommendations for journals and publishers

- Follow prospective trial registration guidelines, seeking confirmation of the primary outcome approved by the human research ethics committee.
- Engage in post-publication peer review. Act on credible challenges by getting involved in correspondence, as well as issuing expressions of concern, errata, or corrigenda when discrepancies arise, rather than inaction, following the COPE, ICMJE, and WAME guidelines.
- Mandate data and case report form sharing in accordance with regulations. Support peer reviewers, providing independent reanalysis of shared data before publication.
- Seek reports of research audits and inspections to be published as supplementary material with studies.
- Facilitate balanced rebuttals and updates, publishing prompt responses to reanalyses, avoiding the impression of unduly resisting scrutiny as outlined in the publication asymmetry phenomenon (Box 5.4).

Roles of institutions, funders, and regulators of drugs and devices

- Ethics committees should take responsibility for investigation and correction when deviations from their approved protocol are identified in the published papers.
- Support data sharing, without barriers, to enable timely reanalyses and prevent prolonged disputes. Avoid perceptions of data concealment, aligning with transparency laws (see Box 7.1 for accountability as a research integrity principle).
- Manage conflicts of interest rigorously and make complete disclosures publicly. Avoid perceptions of conflict of interest concealment, seeking enhanced disclosure as required (Box 4.4).
- Strengthen oversight of academic-industry partnerships through robust research governance. Universities and their affiliated academic research organizations should implement independent audits of collaborative projects for compliance with integrity standards. Make independent oversight a part of the contractual obligation when engaging in academic research with commercial companies. Make the audit reports public.
- Implement integrity training and updates for all research staff, including conflict of interest management (Box 4.4).
- Industry funders should ensure transparency in trial conduct and data sharing, recognizing that sponsorship responsibility cannot be delegated.
- Industry funders should engage constructively with post-publication reanalyses and corrections, as ongoing accountability extends beyond regulatory approval.
- Regulators of drugs and devices should make reports of regulatory inspections public for transparency.
- The case report form should be sought by regulators as part of the documents assessed during drug and device approval.
- Case report forms should be made public in the regulatory documents released, redacted appropriately for privacy protection without obscuring clinical data.
- The data sharing responsibility should be applied equally to all trials, whether or not drug or device regulatory approval is involved.
- To ensure robust follow-up after giving approval, regulators of drugs and devices should include restorations of the originally evaluated trials as part of the post-authorization evidence portfolio.
- Post-publication, actively respond to concerns and participate in the investigation of allegations of research misconduct or questionable practices, promptly correcting the scientific record if required.

Case report form: A paper-based or electronic document used for data collection from each consenting participant in clinical research.

Research governance: The system set up by institutions to oversee that the conduct of research under their auspices is in compliance with regulations.

Audit: A planned formal evaluation of research conduct, i.e. activities (e.g., informed consent), and documents (e.g., data collection and recording), to independently determine if the study is compliant with its approved protocol and meets professional standards such as Good Clinical Practice in human clinical research (GCP).

Inspection: An audit conducted by an external legally competent authority, e.g., a regulator of drugs and devices.

6 *Spinout roller coaster*

Technology transfer in Washington

Technology transfer, the commercialization of academic research and innovation through university spinout companies, offers societal benefits but also amplifies risks when foundational scientific work raises integrity concerns. A Washington State University spinout, founded in 2011, stemmed from doctoral research and won competitive research National Institutes of Health grants. The company's reported value rose rapidly amid high expectations for novel drug development. However, in 2021, post-publication peer review comments led to formal notices of expressions of concern about possible image manipulation in the *Journal of Pharmacology and Experimental Therapeutics*. Subsequent investigations were followed by a cascade of events, including the resignation of the company's co-founder and CEO, and article retractions. Multimillion-dollar settlements resolved (without admission of liability) allegations of undisclosed concerns in research grant applications and alleged misleading disclosures to investors. There was a reported decline in the company's commercial value and a reduction in its workforce. This chapter examines how early-stage academic integrity issues can cascade through technology transfer, research grant funding, and market confidence, offering lessons for the research ecosystem bridging academia and industry.

Research integrity: Undertaking research and publication following ethical and professional principles and standards. Responsible research and publication practices pave the way for science to be regarded as trustworthy. Integrity failures may result from honest errors or deliberate misconduct.

Institution: An academic organization, typically a university, where research takes place. It has the responsibility to oversee ethical and professional research conduct.

Technology transfer

Technology transfer is the process of moving academic research toward commercial application; for example, via licensing research discoveries and inventions to spinout companies. This transfer from universities or research institutions to the private sector turns innovative ideas into practical products and services to benefit society and generate economic returns. Spinout companies are new, independent businesses to which the universities typically transfer or license intellectual property rights concerning a particular technology or research developed within their laboratories. The new company, with its own management team and employees, engages in further research, development, and commercialization. This way, the universities can potentially earn revenue through equity stakes or royalties without being distracted from their core mission of education and basic research.

Typically, a spinout is launched as a private company at a time when the basic research has achieved sufficient maturity to be able to make sustainable progress toward commercialization. The com-

Spinout (spin-off) company: A new, independent business entity formed from a university to commercialize its research.

Funder: Organizations such as government agencies, philanthropists, research charities, industry, etc. that provide funding for research studies or syntheses under contract to institutions.

DOI: 10.1201/9781003655916-6

mercialization tipping point is achieved by providing the proof of principle in real-world conditions, moving stepwise from basic to applied research. For achieving this, companies can bid for funding by making research grant applications to governmental agencies. These tend to be competitive schemes. The grant applications with the most promising foundational scientific works leading to the proposal have the highest chance of success. Peer review of grants relies heavily on the perceived strength and credibility of the references cited to develop the proposal. Successfully funded projects allow development toward a shift in focus from applied research to fully developed commercial systems.

When there is promising progress, the spinout private companies can move towards raising funds via the stock market; for example, through an initial public offering (IPO), selling newly issued shares to investors for the first time to raise capital for growth and expansion. The IPO process is robust, involving filing registration statements with regulatory bodies and marketing roadshows to investors. Foundational scientific data are publicly disclosed to allow securities regulators and investors to assess the company's value, risks, and prospects. Ongoing reporting of the clinical research status is also a critical obligation. Thus, research integrity is a key element of compliance with the securities regulations.

The translation journey from the laboratory bench to successful commercialization is tough. A high proportion of spinout companies fail due to a combination of scientific and financial hurdles. This chapter will explore these dynamics, highlighting how research integrity safeguards are critical. Responsible research practice throughout, from foundational research to grant applications and public disclosures, is not merely an ethical and professional requirement; it is an essential ingredient in securing and sustaining funding and success in both competitive grant awards and public market access.

Basic research: Motivated by curiosity, basic research aims to generate new knowledge.

Applied research: Motivated by the desire to be useful in solving real-world problems, applied research aims to provide solutions.

Initial public offering (IPO): The first time that a private company sells shares of its stock to the public on a stock exchange to raise capital.

Security: Investments, such as stocks, bonds, etc., that are sold to investors by corporations and governments to raise capital.

Box 6.1 Timeline of research integrity concerns: A case study of alleged image manipulation and technology transfer in Washington

Dates	Brief overview of events
2011–13	**Doctoral degree award and publications** Doctoral degree was awarded and the work was published as peer-reviewed journal articles. A biotechnology company was co-founded by the doctoral student to commercially develop drugs from the academic work. *Source: DOIs: 10.1124/jpet.111.185694; 10.1124/jpet.111.188136; 10.1124/jpet.114.218735.*

2014–21	**Post-publication peer review and award of research grants** Large sums of federal research grants ($15 million) were reportedly awarded to the biotechnology company. Several comments concerning the published articles appeared in PubPeer and For Better Science. *Source: URLs: pubpeer.com/publications/51C554512CE22267B2E62172DF3DDE; pubpeer.com/publications/01199F548BE82EE44C7D395568982B; pubpeer.com/publications/D5375331091A7EF887CDC02B813ACA; forbetterscience.com/2021/06/15/how-to-cure-all-diseases; reporter.nih.gov/search/trx0O2fZMUi4YhRJ950y3g/projects; investors.athira.com/news-releases/news-release-details/athira-pharma-awarded-15-million-grant-national-institute-aging; www.geekwire.com/2020/athira-pharma-wins-15m-grant-clinical-trial-alzheimers-drug-national-institute-aging.*
2021	**Expressions of concern** The editors expressed concern about "possible image manipulation after reviewing information received from several sources." They shared these concerns with the corresponding author and their institution. The biotechnology company co-founder was lead author of the articles in question and these had been cited as references in the research grant applications to National Institutes of Health. The co-founder and CEO resigned from the company. The University reportedly removed the doctoral dissertation from its public archive. *Source: DOIs: 10.1124/jpet.111.185694concern; 10.1124/jpet.111.188136concern; 10.1124/jpet.114.218735concern; 10.1124/jpet.112.199497concern. URLs: www.geekwire.com/2021/ex-athira-pharma-ceo-leen-kawas-resigns-leaves-board-image-manipulation-investigation; athirasecuritiessettlement.com/wp-content/uploads/2024/05/0089-_2022-07-29_Order_on_Motion_to_Dismiss.pdf.*
2025	**Retractions** The notices stated that "Following an investigation by Washington State University, Figures … have been found to contain falsified and/or fabricated data." *Source: DOIs: 10.1016/j.jpet.2025.103568; 10.1016/j.jpet.2025.103566; 10.1016/j.jpet.2025.103567.*

2025	**Financial settlements** "The partnership between the scientific community and the federal government is built on trust and shared values of ethical scientific conduct," stated the United States Justice Department when agreeing to a $4,068,698 settlement with the biotechnology company for alleged failure to report allegations of research misconduct to the National Institutes of Health research grant applications. There was a separate settlement of $10,000,000 with affected shareholders. The claims resolved by the settlement were allegations only. There had been no determination of liability. *Source: URLs: athirasecuritiessettlement.com; www.justice.gov/archives/opa/pr/athira-pharma-inc-agrees-pay-4m-settle-false-claims-act-allegations-related-scientific; www.geekwire.com/2025/seattle-biotech-firm-athira-pharma-will-pay-4m-to-settle-allegations-related-to-research-misconduct.*

See Box 6.2 for an outline of the research integrity roles of various actors in this case study and disclaimer. Sources listed above are a few of the many that have covered this case study. This box summarizes reported allegations and findings; no judgment is intended.

A case of a spinout roller coaster

This case study summarizes information from publicly available court records, published retraction notices, and peer-reviewed publications, and discusses them in the context of research integrity scholarship.

In 2011, Washington State University was not ranked in the top 500 of the Shanghai Academic Ranking of World Universities. That year, a doctoral student obtained her PhD degree in molecular pharmacology and co-founded a biotechnology company as a spinout. In the following years, the doctoral work was published in peer-reviewed journals. The *Journal of Pharmacology and Experimental Therapeutics*, with an impact factor of around 4 in 2011, had published the papers. It ranked in Q1 quartile in the pharmacology and pharmacy category (Box 6.1). The journal publisher was Elsevier, which is reported to be one of the world's largest publishers of scientific, technical, and medical literature with over 2500 academic journals. The papers were referenced in grant applications made to the National Institutes of Health, a United States federal government agency for conducting and supporting biomedical and public health research. The company was awarded funding ($15 million) through competitive grants for clinical trials to develop new drugs. In 2020, the private biotechnology spinout became a public company on the stock market through an IPO.

Shanghai ranking: Academic Ranking of World Universities, one of the most influential global research-based university rankings.

Impact factor: A journal statistic dividing the mean number of citations per article in a year by the total number of citable articles published in the previous two years.

Journal quartiles: A journal metric based on citation performance (e.g., impact factor, CiteScore, etc.) ranking all journals in a field into four equal groups, Q1–Q4.

Allegations of image manipulation in the papers and dissertation authored by the company co-founder first appeared on PubPeer, an online platform for post-publication peer review, as early as 2014, with further comments in subsequent years (Box 6.2). These concerns gained public prominence in 2021 following media coverage. The *Journal of Pharmacology and Experimental Therapeutics* issued various expressions of concern and passed the matter on to the university for investigation. The company initiated an independent investigation. Its share price declined significantly, and a class action lawsuit was filed by shareholders alleging violations of federal securities laws through possible omissions or misstatements in the registration statement and other public filings related to its IPO to sell shares on the stock exchange. As the investigations into whether images had been altered in the doctoral dissertation and related papers progressed, the company co-founder resigned as CEO. The company stated publicly that the alterations predated the company's formation and occurred during doctoral work at Washington State University. Court filings in the securities litigation noted that the university had removed the dissertation from its public archive at the end of 2021.

PubPeer: An online platform for post-publication peer review.

Expression of concern: A note published by a journal to inform readers of there being the possibility of a concern about the integrity of a paper.

Box 6.2 Snapshot: The dimensions of research integrity issues in the case study of alleged image manipulation and technology transfer in Washington

Actors and their research integrity roles (described without assessing their adequacy or compliance with standards)	**Reported observations over case study timeline** (no causal inference implied)
Institution: Washington State University	
• Responsibility for overseeing research conduct of its staff and students, including the supervision provided. • Responsible for investigating allegations of research misconduct under its published procedures.	• Multiple retracted articles. • University's Shanghai ranking increased.
Journal: *Journal of Pharmacology and Experimental Therapeutics* belongs to the American Society for Pharmacology and Experimental Therapeutics and published by Elsevier	

• As the journal publishing the articles in question, it had responsibility to peer review the submitted manuscripts before publication. • Following post-publication peer review comments, it passed on the matter to the university for investigation.	• Multiple expressions of concern. • Multiple retracted articles. • Journal impact factor and quartile ranking unchanged.
Industry: A biotechnology company	
• Responsible for preparing grant applications with integrity. • Accountable for conducting itself within federal research and financial securities regulations. • Had responsibility to prepare an accurate research prospectus for investors.	• Settled $4 million in compensation. • Co-founder and CEO resigned. • Market value decreased • Made a separate $10 million settlement with shareholders.
Funder: United states National Institutes of Health	
• Responsible for organizing peer review of research grant applications received for integrity assessment before award. • Had responsibility to pursue grantees where allegations of research integrity concerns are raised.	• Awarded research grants to the biotechnology company. • Received $4 million in settlement.
Sleuthing	
• Sleuths made comments on PubPeer. • Retraction Watch and others blogged on the story.	• Blogs and news stories published.

See Box 1.1 for research integrity terminology.
See Box 1.2 for how research integrity concerns might arise and Box 1.3 for an outline of a research misconduct investigation.
See Box 6.1 for sources of information and the timeline of the case study.
Disclaimer: All factual statements are drawn from published literature and public records. No new allegation of research misconduct, dishonesty, or malice is intended or implied. The case study summarizes publicly available information and does not purport to determine liability or responsibility beyond what has been established in the cited records. References to individuals or organizations are made for academic discussion only and do not attribute intent or fault beyond the public record. When reporting changes in individual, institutional, organizational, and journal status or metrics, no causal inference is implied. The commentary and any opinions expressed are offered in good faith on matters of public interest concerning research integrity. Readers are encouraged to consult the original sources for full context.
University ranking data source: URL: www.shanghairanking.com/rankings/arwu/#### (year).
Journal impact factor and ranking are based on Journal Citation Reports.

In 2025, the journal retracted three papers. A year earlier, the securities class action was resolved through a $10 million settlement, without any admission of liability by the defendants. The National Institutes of Health also pursued a case alleging violation of the False Claims Act based on failure to disclose the research integrity concerns when referencing the papers with possible image manipulation in the research grant applications. The company entered into a settlement agreement with the United States Department of Justice, agreeing to pay $4,068,698 to resolve these allegations, again without admitting liability or wrongdoing. A part of this settlement was paid to a private citizen for their role as a whistleblower assisting the government in recovery. Government officials noted that the company's immediate notification once its board became aware of the issues helped mitigate potential penalties. There was a decline in the company's market capitalization from post-IPO highs associated with substantial workforce reductions (Box 6.3).

This sequence of events underscores several key principles in research integrity and technology transfer. Without implying fault, given that the settlements involved no admissions of liability, the case serves as an instructive example of how transparency obligations can extend across academic, government, and investor contexts in biotechnology. The company, after its humble beginning, had raised over $200 million and was worth over $1 billion at its peak, with investors excited about its promising drug ideas. After research integrity problems came to light involving allegations that its former co-founder altered research images in her doctoral thesis work, the stock price declined substantially (no causal relationship is asserted or implied). The company reportedly implemented substantial workforce reductions as its value shrank to around $25 million in 2025.

In 2025, the company had agreed to pay a $4 million government settlement over allegedly not disclosing the allegations of research integrity issues in research grant applications. A year earlier, after its investors filed a securities class action alleging omissions related to research integrity concerns in IPO disclosures, it settled for $10 million to compensate affected shareholders. The allegations regarding image manipulation were central to the events that led to the settlements, which were resolved without admission of wrongdoing. Washington State University's ranking in the Shanghai Academic Ranking of World Universities in 2025 was in the 401–500 band. As of 2025, the university's former doctoral student had an *h*-index of 9, according to Google Scholar. The Journal of Pharmacology and Experimental Therapeutics impact factor was around 4, and it ranked in Q1 quartile in the pharmacology and pharmacy category. Changes in institutional

Retraction: Removing a published paper from the research record due, for example, to the discovery of a flaw in its integrity.

False Claims Act: Law prohibiting individuals or companies from knowingly submitting false or fraudulent claims for payment to the government.

Market capitalization: The value of a public company traded on the stock market, calculated by multiplying the total number of shares by the share price.

h(Hirsh)-index: A popular statistic to measure scientific output, taking account of citations, e.g., an *h*-index of 5 means that the author has five published papers that have been cited 5 times or more.

Google Scholar: A freely accessible web search engine that indexes scholarly literature across a wide range of formats and disciplines, aggregating nearly all major scholarly publishing.

rankings, academic indices, journal metrics, or market capitalization are reported descriptively only; no causal relationship with the case study is asserted or implied.

Box 6.3 Research integrity concerns, financial settlements, and market capitalization fluctuations of a biotechnology company

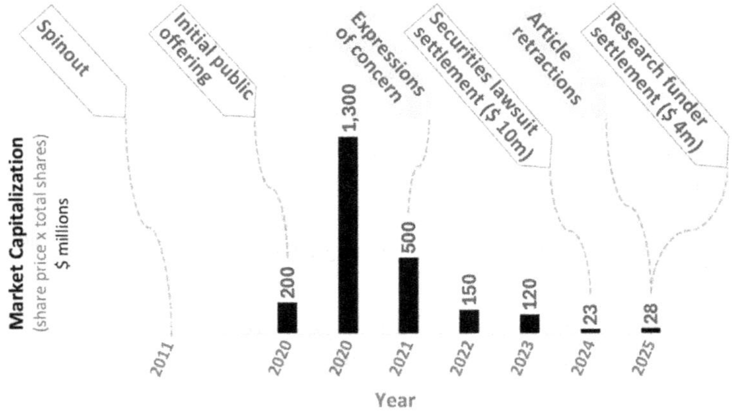

The data presented are approximate.
See Box 6.1 for sources of events in the timeline and Box 6.2 for the disclaimer.
Market capitalization data source: URL: www.macrotrends.net/stocks/charts/ATHA/athira-pharma/market-cap.
When reporting changes in market capitalization, no causal inference is asserted or implied.

Disclosure of research integrity concerns

Drawing from the public records and settlements summarized above, the following analysis reflects on the systemic vulnerabilities in technology transfers.

This case study highlights many systemic vulnerabilities. It highlights the role of sleuths and academic media platforms like PubPeer in surfacing integrity issues. Lessons can be learned concerning various aspects, including the importance of institutional vigilance in technology transfer from academia to industry, the impact of early-career research conduct on commercial ventures years later, the role of disclosure of known concerns in research grant applications with respect to liability, and the value of an accurate scientific prospectus in protecting companies from securities claims by investors.

There is much emphasis in academia on commercialization nowadays. This case underscores the essential role of research integrity as a key principle in research translation. Without implying fault, given that the settlements involved no admissions of liability, the case

Transparency in research: Open research practices including prospective registration, adherence to study design, *a priori* statistical analysis plan, data sharing, timely and complete public reporting, conflict of interest disclosure, open research assessment, open publication practice, etc.

serves as an instructive example of how transparency obligations can extend across academic, governmental, and investor contexts in biotechnology transfer and commercialization. Timely disclosure of known or suspected issues in research grant applications and commercial ventures is highly relevant for spinouts. They rely on attracting external funding to support development and progress from the proof-of-concept stage. Investors may independently assess research integrity as blogs and comments online can be captured via monitoring tools, e.g., the PubPeer platform offers a browser extension or plugin that notifies of potential integrity issues about research cited on webpages. For spinouts reliant on external funding, timely disclosure of any questions regarding foundational science is essential for regulatory compliance. As ventures progress from proof-of-concept to public offerings, the standards for honest and complete reporting intensify. Research integrity forms the vital bridge between scientific research and legal duties to provide truthful information to funders and investors.

Sleuthing: Investigation of possible research and publication misconduct and questionable research practices by volunteer researchers.

Securities regulator: A formal body or agency set up by the government for independent oversight in financial markets.

Box 6.4 Technology transfer and research integrity: Transparency in research and compliance with securities regulations

Scientific credibility

- Investors rely on research conducted and published integrity to believe that an intervention's clinical data and mechanism of action are scientifically valid. Concerns about research misconduct can lead to the collapse of a company's valuation and investor trust.

Requirements

- **Materiality and disclosure:** The securities regulations require companies to disclose all information that a reasonable investor would consider important in making an investment decision (material information). If this underlying information is not trustworthy, the entire prospectus could be considered misleading.
- **Anti-fraud provisions:** The securities regulations prohibit making untrue statements of material fact or omitting material facts. If research harbors suspected fabrication or alteration (e.g., image manipulation), the company and its executives can face severe penalties.

- **Data integrity as a core value:** The drug and device regulators emphasize that data integrity is fundamental to ensuring product safety and efficacy, which in turn forms the basis of trust with authorities. A public company's business is fundamentally dependent on maintaining this trust. ALCOA-CCEA (Attributable, Legible, Contemporaneous, Original, Accurate, Complete, Consistent, Enduring, and Available) framework provides a relevant standard. The elements of the acronym particularly applicable to research integrity in technology transfer include: originality (scientific data from the primary research is required for authenticity in patents, grants, initial public offerings, etc.); accuracy (scientific findings presented must be free from errors and truthful, something that is at the core of all grant proposals and securities disclosures as lapses risk liability); and completeness (full disclosure is mandatory in research grant applications and securities filings; no omissions).

Consequence of failure

- The information shared must be accurate and not misleading. If a company includes data that was generated through unethical or unprofessional research, it may face enforcement actions for fraud.

Source: DOI: 10.1007/s43441-025-00870-3.

Chapter 6: Spinout roller coaster: Technology transfer in Washington – Key points

Advice for researchers

- Maintain rigorous data integrity, avoiding any form of manipulation, such as altering images or reusing data across experiments (see also Chapter 7 for a case study of alleged image manipulation).
- The research integrity of master's and doctoral dissertations is equally important.
- Proactively self-correct and report issues. Acknowledge and address errors early rather than concealing them. Delayed disclosure can lead to amplified fallout.
- Recognize that research conduct in early career can have long-term consequences, particularly when foundational work becomes the basis for spinout companies, grant funding, and public investment.
- Engage in whistleblowing when necessary. If research and publication misconduct or questionable practices are suspected, report promptly in writing to relevant bodies, e.g., institutions, funders, or journals (Box 1.2).

COPE: Committee on Publication Ethics issues guidance to journals on responsible publication practices, including handling research misconduct allegations.

ICMJE: International Committee of Medical Journal Editors provides guidance to journals on publishing policies, such as public prospective registration, data sharing, conflict of interest declaration, etc.

Recommendations for journals and publishers

- Implement advanced detection tools in peer review. Use forensic software to identify image manipulations during submission (also see Chapter 7).
- Accelerate expression of concern and retraction processes. Act swiftly on post-publication allegations, e.g., via platforms like PubPeer, to limit the downstream impact of potentially flawed papers.
- Foster transparency in corrections, issuing clear expressions of concern or retraction notices to maintain scientific trust.
- When expressions of concern or retractions involve foundational research that has been cited in grant applications or used to support commercialization, notify relevant funders and institutional technology transfer offices to enable coordinated responses.
- In cases of retractions associated with research integrity concerns, conduct root cause analyses to examine vulnerabilities in the peer review process and editor accountability, and to determine the need for training initiatives.

Roles of institutions and funders

- Strengthen oversight of academic-industry partnerships. Universities and their affiliated academic research organizations should independently audit collaborative projects for compliance with integrity standards. Make independent oversight a part of the contractual obligation when engaging in academic research with commercial companies.
- Implement research integrity training and updates so that early-career researchers develop awareness of the cascading consequences of any flaws in foundational research in subsequent spinout companies, grant funding, and public market confidence (Box 7.1).
- Implement technology transfer oversight that includes integrity verification before commercialization.
- Establish clear policies requiring disclosure of research integrity concerns in grant applications and technology transfer documents. Failure to disclose known or suspected issues can result in False Claims Act liability and securities law violations.
- Manage conflicts of interest rigorously and make declarations publicly (Box 4.4).
- Post-publication, actively participate in the investigation of allegations and promptly correct the scientific record if required (Box 1.3).

WAME: World Association of Medical Editors. It aims to improve editorial standards through self-regulation.

Accountability: A responsible research principle guiding individuals and organizations to be answerable for the research they engage in from idea to post-publication.

Research culture: The academic environment comprising the norms, values, expectations, attitudes, and behaviors within research organizations. Academic freedom, collegiality, collaboration, equality and diversity, research integrity (ethics and professionalism), conflict management with openness, accountability, and transparency are all features of the research culture.

- Spinout companies should ensure that research integrity due diligence is conducted before IPOs and other public offerings. Securities regulations require disclosure of material information, including research integrity concerns that could affect investor decisions (Box 6.4).
- Funders should implement mechanisms to identify and act on research integrity concerns that emerge after grants are awarded, including the ability to recover funds where misconduct is found.

7 *All that glitters may not be gold*

Image manipulation and resignation in Stanford

Accountability, as a core virtue of research integrity, refers to the obligation of researchers and organizations to answer for every aspect of their work. All their actions and decisions in the conduct and publication of their research are covered, including upholding standards and accepting responsibility in case there are failures to meet them. In a high-profile case involving a senior academic leader at Stanford University, an independent investigation confirmed data manipulation in papers published in top-tier journals and a pattern of failing to correct the scientific record. Across multiple institutions, the work undertaken exhibited an "unusual frequency" of "data manipulation" over many years. The independent panel concluded this pattern indicated a failure to foster a culture of integrity, reinforcing the principle that ultimate responsibility for a research group's conduct falls on its leader. While the inquiry found no evidence of the senior scientist's personal involvement in "image manipulations," it highlighted a critical deficit in the fulfillment of accountability as a leader. There were retractions of papers in top peer-reviewed journals, including *Cell*, *Science*, and *Nature*. This chapter analyzes the case study to explore how accountability mechanisms function or fail when applied to individuals at the highest echelons of academic research, and what this reveals about the stewardship of integrity in elite scientific institutions.

Research integrity: Undertaking research and publication following ethical and professional principles and standards. Responsible research and publication practices pave the way for science to be regarded as trustworthy. Integrity failures may result from honest errors or deliberate misconduct.

Scientific virtue: A character trait or a disposition to consistently act in a manner that will best achieve research excellence.

Accountability as a scientific virtue

A scientific virtue is a character trait describing a disposition to consistently act in a manner that is likely to best achieve excellence. Scientific progress relies fundamentally on trust in the integrity of the research record. This trust is sustained by a framework of ethical and professional norms, among which accountability stands as a paramount virtue. Within research integrity, accountability refers to the principle that individual researchers and institutions must be answerable for the conduct, oversight, and outcomes of their scientific work. It encompasses the duty of researchers to ensure the validity or accuracy of their data, to provide transparent methodology, to credit contributions accurately, etc., and, crucially, to correct the record when errors are identified. For research leaders, this virtue extends

Institution: An academic organization, typically a university, where research takes place. It has the responsibility to oversee ethical and professional research conduct.

DOI: 10.1201/9781003655916-7

beyond personal research conduct and includes a responsibility for the research environment they cultivate and the work undertaken and published under their authority.

Research integrity codes consistently articulate an ideal of accountability that is both individual and organizational, e.g., ALLEA or ALL European Academies has issued a code built upon four overarching principles, including reliability, honesty, respect, and accountability. Leadership in research carries a heightened dimension of this accountability. Senior scientists in positions of authority are entrusted not only with advancing knowledge but also with stewarding the integrity culture of their laboratories and institutions. Their actions or inactions in addressing or ignoring integrity concerns within their own research groups send a powerful signal about institutional values. When accountability is fully realized, it reinforces a self-correcting scientific process and models responsible behavior for trainees, mentees, and colleagues. When it is neglected, it can undermine confidence in entire fields and institutions.

Some key elements of accountability as a research integrity principle include answerability, responsible readership, duty of correction, consequence acceptance, and transparency (Box 7.1). Cultivation of these elements in the research culture should be an organizational objective. Accountability is codified as a non-negotiable pillar of ethical and professional research, yet its practical enforcement remains one of the most contentious challenges in research governance. Extending beyond the individual research employees working under institutional oversight, it covers the integrity of the published record. The application of this integrity principle becomes profoundly strained when the subject of scrutiny is not a budding scholar in a mediocre university publishing in an unremarkable journal but an esteemed leader of a premier university with high-profile outputs in top-tier journals. In this situation, reputation and authority cast a long shadow over the accountability mechanisms. This chapter looks at a case study for analyzing how the principle of accountability is interpreted, applied, and enforced when concerns arise about the work of individuals at the pinnacle of the academic hierarchy publishing in top-tier journals, testing the resilience of integrity systems designed to uphold this fundamental virtue. The health of the scientific ecosystem depends on ensuring that the weight of accountability is not inversely proportional to the stature of the researchers, institutions, and journals it must bind.

Accountability: A responsible research principle guiding individuals and organizations to be answerable for the research they engage in from idea to post-publication.

ALLEA (ALL European Academies): European federation of academies of sciences and humanities.

Organization: Any entity, be it an institution, funder, university, hospital, publisher, regulator, etc., that is a legally constituted body to undertake a function.

Research culture: The academic environment comprising the norms, values, expectations, attitudes, and behaviors within research organizations. Academic freedom, collegiality and collaboration, equality and diversity, research integrity (ethics and professionalism), conflict management with openness, accountability, and transparency are all features of the research culture.

Box 7.1 Accountability as a research integrity principle

Accountability feature	Comments
Answerability	The obligation to provide transparent, timely explanations for research decisions, methods, results, and conclusions.
Oversight and supervision	The duty to actively monitor and ensure the integrity of all research conducted under one's authority, including the supervision and mentoring of team members and colleagues.
Stewardship of the research record	The responsibility to ensure the accuracy, completeness, and honest presentation of all data, figures, and findings, enabling verification.
Duty of correction	The affirmative obligation to identify, disclose, and formally correct errors or misleading information in the scientific record.
Transparency	The proactive disclosure of methodologies, data (including raw data where possible), conflicts of interest, funding sources, and any limitations or uncertainties in the research.
Consequence acceptance	The willingness to accept reasonable professional or institutional repercussions for possible failures to uphold integrity standards. Seeking forgiveness after the event in the form of an apology alone is not a substitute for accountability.
Cultivation of an integrity culture	The responsibility of leaders to foster an environment that prioritizes ethics, professionalism, openness, and rigor over producing positive results.

See Chapters 2, 10, and 12 for more case studies emphasizing accountability as a research integrity principle.
See Box 4.4 for conflict of interest management.
Source: DOI: 10.1007/pl00022268. URLs: allea.org/wp-content/uploads/2023/06/European-Code-of-Conduct-Revised-Edition-2023.pdf; ori.hhs.gov/sites/default/files/rcrintro.pdf.

A case study of accountability in default

Impact factor: A journal statistic dividing the mean number of citations per article in a year by the total number of citable articles published in the previous two years.

In 2016, Stanford University was ranked second to the top of the Shanghai Academic Ranking of World Universities. That year, some past papers of its new president came under criticism on the PubPeer academic online platform as part of post-publication peer review (Box 7.2). The papers had originally been published in top peer-reviewed journals *Cell*, *Science*, and *Nature* in the years 1999–2009. At the time of publication, the journals *Cell*, *Science*, and *Nature*, respectively, had impact factors of 36 (ranked in Q1 quartile in the cell biology and biochemistry category), 23, and 31 (both ranked in Q1 quartile in the multidisciplinary category). Note that *Science* and *Nature* are the journals that the Shanghai Academic Ranking of World Universities recognizes as world-class on account of their rigorous peer review and selection processes. Publication in these two journals is viewed as a mark of groundbreaking research, and the ranking methodology recognizes this as a defining characteristic of a top-tier research university. To even be in a position to be considered for the Shanghai ranking, a university must have at least one paper published in *Science* or *Nature*; other entry criteria include having a Nobel Prize or Field Medal winner or a highly cited researcher.

The 2015–2016 PubPeer comments were mainly by anonymous platform users who posted detailed analyses pointing to apparent image manipulations in several high-impact papers from the laboratory led by the senior scientist who was now the Stanford University president. By 2016, the four *Cell*, *Science* (two papers), and *Nature* papers in question, which were ultimately retracted, had been cited around 700, 600, 250, and 900 times, respectively, according to Google Scholar. There was no official expression of concern issued by the journals, according to bibliometric searches. In fact, the authors had approached *Cell* and *Science*, but the former declined to publish a correction, and the latter failed to publish the correction due to a journal error. There was a second wave of PubPeer criticisms in 2022. The PubPeer posts represented a modern post-publication peer review function in the digital age. They may be regarded as part of the scientific community's effort to police the scientific record in a new way that is decentralized, not controlled by journals publishing the articles in the same old manner as their letters and correspondence sections had done in the past. The initial 2016 comments had elicited no public response from the authors, their affiliated institutions, or the journals. The second time in 2022, however, some journals issued expressions of concern, and the university initiated an independent investigation of the allegations of research misconduct.

In 2023, the independent panel issued its 95-page research misconduct investigation report. It confirmed the core allegations and identified deeper systemic failures. The independent investigation report concluded that the Stanford University president did not personally commit any research fraud; however, the laboratory he led as a senior scientist exhibited a pattern of research integrity failures. The panel found evidence of data manipulation necessitating retractions or corrections. Critically, the report documented a repeated failure to uphold the duty of scientific record correction, with multiple ignored opportunities. The report attributed these failures to a research culture that lacked rigor and to inadequate oversight, as there appeared

PubPeer: An online platform for post-publication peer review.

Shanghai ranking: Academic Ranking of World Universities, one of the most influential global research-based university rankings.

Journal quartiles: A journal metric based on citation performance (e.g., impact factor, CiteScore, etc.) ranking all journals in a field into four equal groups, Q1–Q4.

Expression of concern: A note published by a journal to inform readers of there being the possibility of a concern about the integrity of a paper.

Sleuthing: Investigation of possible research and publication misconduct and questionable research practices by volunteer researchers.

to be a long reluctance to correct errors. The panel's central finding was one of leadership and accountability failure. The panel did not find that individual acts of data manipulation were on the part of the senior scientist. In response to the report, he resigned from the university presidency. Observations based on the public record over the two-decade timeline, from original publication to PubPeer comments to the president's resignation, serve as a roadmap of accountability in default with potential for long-lasting reputational damage.

Retraction: Removing a published paper from the research record due, for example, to the discovery of a flaw in its integrity.

Box 7.2 Timeline of research integrity concerns: A case study of alleged accountability failure in Stanford

Dates	Brief overview of events
1999–2009	**Original publications** *Cell*, *Science*, and *Nature* publications. *Sources: DOIs: 10.1016/s0092-8674(00)80804-1; 10.1126/science.1058445; 10.1126/science.1059391; 10.1038/nature03080; 10.1038/nature07767.*
2015–16	**First post-publication peer review comments** Initial comments concerning the published articles appeared in PubPeer. *Sources: URLs: pubpeer.com/publications/250D42FBB7D7298E704BFD6CD8B22A; pubpeer.com/publications/B6410F2AF1398E6F379B244E7520A1; pubpeer.com/publications/59C3359E71EED451E01AF46CFDC0BC; pubpeer.com/publications/BFCF07AC5A957DB7E8950B448CB6CB.*
2022	**Second wave of post-publication peer review comments and expressions of concern** A set of follow-up comments and a new comment appeared on PubPeer. Grassroots journalism provided the pressure for the university to undertake formal investigation. At this stage, journals also issued expressions of concern. In one of these, the journal *Cell* stated that in 2015 it had declined to publish a correction due to its polices at the time; a decision that was reversed by the retraction later on. In two of these, the authors had provided corrected images in 2015, but the journal *Science* stated that it never posted an erratum due to an error. *Sources: DOIs: 10.1016/j.cell.2022.12.019; 10.1126/science.adg2860; 10.1126/science.adg2852. URLs: www.highereddive.com/news/stanford-university-investigates-its-president-over-research-misconduct-acc/637633; /stanforddaily.com/2022/11/29/stanford-presidents-research-under-investigation-for-scientific-misconduct-university-admits-mistakes; pubpeer.com/publications/467FA67858F959040F2EABE876A7B3.*

2023	**Independent investigation report and resignation** A 95-page investigation report made public showed multiple examples of "data manipulation" occurring at an "unusual frequency" at different times at different institutions. The independent panel observed that the lead researcher "took inadequate steps to correct mistakes in the scientific record." The report did not find that the senior researcher subject of the investigation "had actual intent or knowledge or was reckless as to any research misconduct." The report stated that "science in general could benefit from a deeper recognition by senior scientists that they need to be mindful to defuse any putative pressure to please a Principal Investigator beyond the significant, ordinary pressure that postdocs already experience in a competitive scientific field." *Sources: URLs: boardoftrustees.stanford.edu/sites/g/files/sbiybj31576/files/media/file/scientific-panel-final-report.pdf; stanforddaily.com/2023/02/17/internal-review-found-falsified-data-in-stanford-presidents-alzheimers-research-colleagues-allege; www.science.org/content/article/stanford-president-to-step-down-despite-probe-exonerating-him-of-research-misconduct; www.nytimes.com/2023/07/19/us/stanford-president-resigns-tessier-lavigne.html.*
2023–26	**Retractions and expressions of concern** Four 1999–2009 papers were retracted and two had expressions of concern issued.*Sources: DOIs: 10.1016/j.cell.2023.08.024; 10.1126/science.adk1517; 10.1126/science.adk1521; 10.1038/s41586-023-06944-2; 10.1038/s41586-023-06943-3; 10.1038/44521; 10.1038/s41586-025-10080-4. URL: retractionwatch.com/2023/12/18/former-stanford-president-retracts-nature-paper-as-another-gets-expression-of-concern.*

See Box 7.3 for an outline of the research integrity roles of various actors in this case study and disclaimer. Sources listed above are a few of the many that have covered this case study. This box summarizes reported allegations and findngs; no judgment is intended.

The scientist's resignation was associated with the retraction of four papers and two expressions of concern during 2023–2026. When the *Cell*, *Science* (two papers), and *Nature* papers were ultimately retracted, they had already accrued over 900, 700, 300, and 1300 citations, respectively, according to Google Scholar, i.e., over 750 more citations since 2016 when the concerns were first raised publicly. In 2025, the university had new leadership. Its ranking in the Academic Ranking of World Universities had remained unchanged (Box 7.3). The university's former president had an *h*-index of 158 on Google Scholar at the time of writing this book. The journals *Cell*, *Science*, and *Nature*,

h(Hirsh)-index: A popular statistic to measure scientific output, taking account of citations, e.g., an *h*-index of 5 means that the author has 5 published papers that have been cited 5 times or more.

respectively, had impact factors of 42 (ranked in Q1 quartile in the cell biology and biochemistry category), 57, and 48 (both ranked in Q1 quartile in the multidisciplinary category) in 2025. *Science* and *Nature* journals remain part of the Shanghai Academic Ranking of World Universities. Changes in institutional rankings, academic indices, or journal metrics are reported descriptively only; no causal relationship with the case study is asserted or implied.

Google Scholar: A freely accessible web search engine that indexes scholarly literature across a wide range of formats and disciplines, aggregating nearly all major scholarly publishing.

Box 7.3 Snapshot: The dimensions of research integrity issues in the case study of alleged accountability failure in Stanford

Actors and their research integrity roles (described without assessing their adequacy or compliance with standards)	**Reported observations over case study timeline** (no causal inference implied)
Institution: Stanford University	
• Responsibility for overseeing research conduct of its staff and research groups. • Responsible for investigating allegations of research misconduct under its published procedures.	• Multiple retracted articles and expressions of concern. • University's Shanghai ranking unchanged. • Resignation of university president.
Journals: *Cell*, *Science*, and *Nature* published by Elsevier, American Association for the Advancement of Science, and Springer Nature, respectively	
• The journal publishing the articles in question had the responsibility to peer review the submitted manuscripts before publication. • Following initial public post-publication peer review comments, two of the journals failed to publish corrections given by authors. • Following repeat public post-publication peer review comments, they responded with expressions of concern and retractions.	• Multiple expressions of concern. • Multiple retracted articles. • Journals' impact factors and quartile rankings unchanged.

Sleuthing

- Sleuths commented on PubPeer and repeated the critique when there was no response by authors, institutions, and journals publicly.
- Grassroot journalism initially covered the story.
- Comments and news stories initially published were picked up by mainstream media.

See Box 1.1 for research integrity terminology.
See Box 1.2 for how research integrity concerns might arise and Box 1.3 for an outline of a research misconduct investigation.
See Box 7.2 for sources of information and the timeline of the case study.
Disclaimer: All factual statements are drawn from published literature and public records. No new allegation of research misconduct, dishonesty, or malice is intended or implied. The case study summarizes publicly available information and does not purport to determine liability or responsibility beyond what has been established in the cited records. References to individuals or organizations are made for academic discussion only and do not attribute intent or fault beyond the public record. When reporting changes in individual, institutional, organizational, and journal status or metrics, no causal inference is implied. The commentary and any opinions expressed are offered in good faith on matters of public interest concerning research integrity. Readers are encouraged to consult the original sources for full context.
University ranking data source: URL: www.shanghairanking.com/rankings/arwu/#### (year).
Journal impact factor and ranking are based on Journal Citation Reports.

Halo effect: Layers of accountability

Drawing from the investigation report and public record summarized above, the following analysis reflects on the systemic factors that may delay accountability.

This case study moves the discussion from the question of whether there was any misconduct and which specific accountabilities were breached to what that tells us about power and integrity in the research ecosystem. The case shows how the normal channels of scientific self-correction can be obstructed by hierarchy, and how true accountability can be achieved when public scrutiny overwhelms organizational inertia, both at the institutional and the journal level. The case study stands as a modern parable: in the digital age, the scientific record with or without any inherent errors is permanently visible, and community scrutiny is persistent; the choice faced is between voluntary, timely, public accountability at the point when the issues come to attention or procrastination associated with eventual, enforced correction.

The delayed and reluctant institutional response to allegations against its president can be understood through the lens of what has been termed the halo effect. Monumental achievements, e.g., an ex-

COPE: Committee on Publication Ethics issues guidance to journals on responsible publication practices, including handling research misconduct allegations.

ICMJE: International Committee of Medical Journal Editors provides guidance to journals on publishing policies, such as public prospective registration, data sharing, conflict of interest declaration, etc.

ceptionally high *h*-index for an individual scientist (see Chapter 2), a premier academic ranking for an institution, or an exceedingly high impact factor for a journal, cast a halo. The bias, where high esteem can color judgment, can make allegations against top-tier scientists, institutions, or journals appear incongruous, potentially affecting both external and internal evaluations of the concerns raised. This situation demands demonstration of adherence to accountability as a research integrity principle (Box 7.1).

WAME: World Association of Medical Editors. It aims to improve editorial standards through self-regulation.

The halo effect describes the external bias that shields those at the top from scrutiny, but there can also be an internal dimension. When isolated from critical feedback, those at the top may develop what some commentators have termed insulated hubris. Self-confidence and pride due to exceptional achievements can generate deference that may lead to criticism being dismissed. Over time, the absence of consequential feedback reinforces a sense of invulnerability, creating an environment where corrective norms are not prioritized. In this background, allegations on PubPeer may not be treated as serious scientific critiques but as nuisances. The failure of authors and editors to publicly respond to the PubPeer comments and lack of follow-up through corrections in journals (on two occasions, the journals attributed the lack of correction to internal errors) shows that normal mechanisms of post-publication scrutiny had become suspended. Oversight responsibility was neglected as the investigation concluded that the "unusual frequency of manipulation of research data … in labs at different institutions" indicated a failure of laboratory supervision. The investigation report's findings highlighted repeated failures in the duty of correction. This violation nullifies the emphasis on honesty and reliability as errors remain uncorrected. Record stewardship was compromised, as original data for old experiments was unavailable or problematic. As the report found, cultivation of an integrity culture was deficient, with the panel noting a lab culture that "lacked rigor" with a failure in the leader's role to model and enforce integrity. Notably, the sole feature where accountability was partially enforced was consequence acceptance, though only after extreme external pressure. Answerability was evaded for over two decades when asked about problematic images. Formal scrutiny occurred only after the persistent, public, and technically detailed critiques on PubPeer, amplified by grassroots journalism, gained significant attention. The case illustrates how accountability mechanisms can falter in a context where individual, institutional, and journal prestige may delay or diminish the perceived urgency of addressing concerns raised about potential integrity flaws.

Transparency in research: Open research practices including prospective registration, adherence to study design, *a priori* statistical analysis plan, data sharing, timely and complete public reporting, conflict of interest disclosure, open research assessment, open publication practice, etc.

This case study of research integrity failures involving a top institution and highly ranked journals is not merely a story of flawed data, but a chronicle of organizational accountability delayed, deferred, and ultimately forced. The timeline of events reveals a stark disconnect between the moment problems became publicly known and the moment they were formally addressed by the institution and journals vested with ultimate oversight. This gap, stretching from 2015 to 2026, is the central feature illustrating how prestige and positional power can insulate serious allegations from timely scrutiny.

Chapter 7: All that glitters may not be gold: Image manipulation and resignation in Stanford – Key points

Advice for researchers

- Cultivate a culture of integrity, not just productivity, with rigorous documentation, open discussion of negative results, and questioning of methods.
- Mentorship must explicitly include training in research ethics and professionalism.
- Proactive correction is a professional duty, not just an optional extra. Addressing errors is a hallmark of integrity.
- Senior scientists in leadership roles offer the final safeguard as they bear non-delegable, ultimate accountability for all data, authorship, and the integrity of publications bearing their name.
- Actively monitor post-publication critique, e.g., on platforms like PubPeer, and engage with correction processes decisively and transparently. Passivity is a breach of accountability (Box 7.1).
- Follow up with journals after offering corrections to ensure that corrigenda are published.
- Sleuth with responsibility but without fear or favor (Box 1.2; also see Chapters 2 and 10).

Recommendations for journals and publishers

- Apply consistent scrutiny regardless of author prestige. Allegations against high-profile authors require the same urgent, rigorous investigation as those against early-career researchers.
- The peer review and post-publication processes must be blind to the halo effect.
- Audit and enforce figure or image integrity proactively. Im-

plement and standardize the use of forensic image screening tools, e.g., Proofig (URL: www.proofig.com), ImageTwin (URL: imagetwin.ai), during manuscript review.

- Move integrity checks of data, including images, approvals, consent, etc., in bulk from a reactive to a preventative stance. Nip the evil in the editorial assessment bud (see Chapters 4, 10, and 12 concerning documentation of human research ethics committee approval as an integrity check).
- Mandate transparent correction pathways, holding corresponding authors accountable for participating in and publicly tracking the status of unresolved allegations.

Halo Effect: Highly prolific or renowned researchers, e.g., Nobel laureates, may be subjected to less scrutiny by journals, peer reviewers, and data sleuths. However, they have earned retractions of their articles, so there is no place for double standards in research integrity assessments.

Role of institutions

- Create clear, confidential, and independent channels for whistleblowing or reporting concerns about senior leaders, insulating the process from institutional politics and reputational self-interest (Box 1.2).
- Establish truly independent investigation pathways (Box 1.3).
- Decouple administrative power from research oversight. Those overseeing integrity investigations into allegations must not report to the subject of the inquiry.
- Governance structures, e.g., the board of trustees' committees, must be empowered and willing to act independently of the administration.
- Define and enforce consequential accountability for leaders, making explicit that leadership positions heighten, rather than diminish, accountability (Box 7.1).
- Sanctions for integrity failures by senior leaders must be meaningful and transparent, helping to build institutional culture on a foundation of rigor and accountability (see Chapter 10).

8 *Alleged misconduct in charity-funded research*

Breach of contract and an investigation in Portsmouth

Research integrity: Undertaking research and publication following ethical and professional principles and standards. Responsible research and publication practices pave the way for science to be regarded as trustworthy. Integrity failures may result from honest errors or deliberate misconduct.

The research ecosystem engages in amplifying new scientific results via social and mainstream media to boost public image. Research integrity failures introduce a serious flaw in this approach, as retraction of the research promoted can bite back. The charitable sector is particularly vulnerable in this regard. Its well-meaning contribution to support science can result in reputational damage in case of findings of research misconduct. This chapter examines the intersection of research misconduct, commercial development, charitable partnership, and contractual liability, as described in published records and court proceedings. It traces the trajectory of a promising breakthrough from its high-profile publication, explicitly acknowledging the support received from various charitable and commercial funders. It follows the 2019 *Cancer Letters* paper, to its eventual retraction in 2021 prompted by findings concerning alleged data irregularities by an institutional investigation. Crucially, as the case becomes entangled in litigation, the high court's judgment offers the opportunity for a dissection of how a breach of contract for failing to undertake and publish research with integrity comes to a settlement with a one-million-pound liability for the claimant's losses. By evaluating the roles of researchers, institutions, journals, and funders, this chapter will provide a framework for due diligence. The case study gives useful advice for research charities to protect themselves against the fallout of the risks associated with research integrity failures that traditional oversight is ill-equipped to manage.

Charitable sector

Organization: Any entity, be it an institution, funder, university, hospital, publisher, regulator, etc., that is a legally constituted body to undertake a function.

The global medical research charity sector represents a vital third pillar of scientific advancement, operating alongside government and commercial industry. Unlike state-led funding, which is often tied to broad public policy, or pharmaceutical investment, which prioritizes commercial viability, medical research charities are driven by patient priorities in the pursuit of solutions for unmet medical needs. They can bridge various gaps at any stage in the entire research translation

DOI: 10.1201/9781003655916-8

journey between basic laboratory discovery and clinical application. Charities vary in size and ambition. They are vulnerable to the difficulties that may arise due to research misconduct, as they tend to operate without the strict research oversight frameworks that funders in government and commercial sectors have. However, nowadays, the role of citizen involvement in research is also creating a more formal place for them on the research planning and delivery tables.

From global giants like the Wellcome Trust and the Bill & Melinda Gates Foundation to niche, disease-specific small charitable organizations, these entities collectively contribute billions annually to the global health research base. On the one hand, the charitable sector can invest in infrastructure, establishing named centers of excellence within universities to foster long-term innovation, and, on the other hand, it can offer small project grants to pump-prime promising but high-risk research that may struggle to attract government grants or private capital. Charities are also increasingly adopting venture philanthropy models, taking part in spinouts (see Chapter 6). Frequently, their fundraising campaigns leverage the results of their own research funding. Whatever the shape or form, the charitable role as a funder of hope carries risks concerning research integrity and institutional oversight. Their reputations become inextricably linked to the integrity of the projects they support, and in turn, this impacts their ability to attract donations.

Even in countries where there are robust frameworks for the regulation of charities, such as the United Kingdom, the sector remains vulnerable to research integrity issues. Over a recent seven-year period, the Wellcome Trust was notified of over 50 allegations of research misconduct according to their annual research integrity reports (URL: wellcome.org/research-funding/guidance/policies-grant-conditions/responsible-conduct-research). In the enthusiasm for their noble mission, charities may overlook the necessity for cold, forensic due diligence. Reliance on institutional oversight without external independent verification can lead to challenges in maintaining research integrity standards. This can create a precarious environment where scientific misconduct and questionable practices do not merely result in retracted papers; they may cause a profound breach of trust with donors and a devastating loss of momentum for patient communities awaiting a cure. This delicate balance between charitable mission and responsibility for scientific rigor was put to the test in a collaboration between a university research institute, a pharmaceutical company, and their charitable partners. What began as a hopeful investment into a novel intervention transformed from a public relations triumph into a cautionary tale of the breakdown of research integrity and insti-

Funder: Organizations such as government agencies, philanthropists, research charities, industry, etc. that provide funding for research studies or syntheses under contract to institutions.

Research translation: Research development from the laboratory bench to the patients' bedside, i.e., moving from basic to applied research.

Basic research: Motivated by curiosity, basic research aims to generate new knowledge.

Applied research: Motivated by the desire to be useful in solving real-world problems, applied research aims to provide solutions.

Institution: An academic organization, typically a university, where research takes place. It has the responsibility to oversee ethical and professional research conduct.

tutional liability. The associated reputational, legal, and financial collapse resonated far beyond the laboratory walls.

A case study of alleged breach of the research contract

Spinout (spin-off) company: A new, independent business entity formed from a university to commercialize its research.

PubPeer: An online platform for post-publication peer review.

Sleuthing: Investigation of possible research and publication misconduct and questionable research practices by volunteer researchers.

This case study summarizes information from PubPeer comments, court documents, retraction notices, peer-reviewed publications, and publicly available companies house records, and discusses them in the context of research integrity scholarship.

A legal dispute between a pharmaceutical company and a university had its origins in a contract to undertake research for the development of a novel pharmaceutical intervention designed to treat a serious disease. The formulation, which would later be marketed under a commercial brand name, was invented by the company's founders. In 2016, an academic-industry partnership was established formally at the University of Portsmouth through an agreement signed under United Kingdom laws. Another party to the agreement was a registered charitable organization. The foundational scientific basis of the collaboration was an unpublished pilot study showing promising results conducted by a staff member of the university to test the potential of the intervention; this work was undertaken a year earlier at the laboratory of another leading research institution. The partnership was established to undertake further rigorous scientific research in a charity-backed university laboratory, with the project funding provided jointly by the company and the charity signatories on the agreement to generate the evidence required for taking the steps toward regulatory approval and commercial scaling.

Box 8.1 Timeline of research integrity concerns: A case study of alleged breach of contract in Portsmouth

Dates	Brief overview of events
2015–16	**Academic-industry partnership** Underpinned by an unpublished pilot study, a contract established an academic-industry partnership for further research with a grant given by the industry partner to the University of Portsmouth with a view to later undertake commercialization. *Source: www.farrer.co.uk/news-and-insights/excluding-liability-for-dishonest-breach-be-careful-what-you-wish-for.*

2019	**Journal peer review, publication, post-publication peer review, and corrigendum** Hailed as a paper "opening the door," a key article was published, acknowledging the financial support of the company, in *Cancer Letters* in May 2019 following peer review. By August 2019, comments highlighting data integrity concerns and author's response had appeared in PubPeer. A corrigendum followed in October 2019. It triggered further PubPeer comments by anonymous users identifying errors, with one stating, "Does this mean we will have a corrigendum to the corrigendum?" For Better Science and Retraction Watch (covering another paper) blogs added to the pressure. *Source: DOIs: 10.1016/j.canlet.2019.05.028; 0.1016/j.canlet.2019.10.002. URLs: www.dailymail.co.uk/news/article-7324913/Brain-tumour-treatment-set-revolutionised-cheap-drug.html; www.port.ac.uk/news-events-and-blogs/news/shrinking-brain-tumours-and-opening-the-door-for-targeted-cancer-therapies; www.sciencedaily.com/releases/2019/08/190805134003.htm; eurekalert.org/news-releases/592558; pubpeer.com/publications/A3CE30841D4D7057101381E55486A3; forbetterscience.com/2019/08/21/richard-hill-the-man-even-gels-are-afraid-of; retractionwatch.com/2019/08/28/i-sincerely-apologise-uk-cancer-specialist-calls-for-retraction-of-his-work-years-after-its-flagged-on-pubpeer.*
2020	**Investigation of research misconduct allegations** The court records show that the university convened a formal disciplinary panel according to its procedure for the investigation of allegations of misconduct in research, involving external experts.
2021	**Retraction** In 2021, the *Cancer Letters* journal retracted the article. The retraction notice stated that the "University concluded their investigation with external experts and determined that misconduct did take place in relation to the research involved in this paper." *Source: DOI:* 10.1016/j.canlet.2019.05.028.
2023-24	**Breach of contract court case and financial settlement** The university was ordered by the court to pay a settlement of £1,000,000 to the pharmaceutical company following a legal dispute regarding a breach of contract, which involved findings related to research conduct. *Source: URLs:* www.bailii.org/ew/cases/EWHC/TCC/2024/35.pdf; *forbetterscience.com/2024/09/16/bushell-on-the-hill-or-legitimate-errors-which-do-crop-into-papers; gowlingwlg.com/en/insights-resources/articles/2024/can-you-exclude-liability-for-dishonesty.*

2025	**Pharmaceutical company liquidation** The company's public records show that it had filed for liquidation (compulsory wind up commencing January 2025). *Source: URL:* https://find-and-update.company-information.service.gov.uk/company/09209053/insolvency.

See Box 8.2 for an outline of the research integrity roles of various actors in this case study, along with the disclaimer.
Sources listed above are a few of the many that have covered this case study. This box summarizes reported allegations and findings; no judgment is intended.

In 2017, the University of Portsmouth was ranked in the Shanghai Academic Ranking of World Universities in the 501–600 band for the first time, having been granted university status in 1992; it had been a polytechnic institute in the United Kingdom since 1960. The research being undertaken as part of the partnership program reached its apparent peak in May 2019 with the publication of a paper in a prominent oncology journal, *Cancer Letters*, owned and published by Elsevier. The publisher is reported to be one of the world's largest publishers of scientific, technical, and medical literature with over 2500 academic journals. The *Cancer Letters* journal impact factor was around 7, and it ranked in Q1 quartile in the cancer research category at the time when the paper was published. The journal offered high visibility to the work as the paper immediately attracted international attention, as its findings suggested that the intervention could offer a new form of treatment for patients with the disease. The paper acknowledged the pharmaceutical company's financial support as well as that of the charitable sector.

Shanghai ranking: Academic Ranking of World Universities, one of the most influential global research-based university rankings.

Impact factor: A journal statistic dividing the mean number of citations per article in a year by the total number of citable articles published in the previous two years.

At the time it was published, the paper was celebrated as a landmark breakthrough, including in the mainstream media. The plan was to progress from there to first-in-human studies. However, the data within the paper soon became the subject of intense scrutiny on the post-publication peer review platform PubPeer (Box 8.1). Sleuths reported data anomalies, including concerns about possible image manipulation. These criticisms intensified in August 2019, as For Better Science and Retraction Watch (covering another paper that got retracted) made further comments. The lead researcher was quick to respond to the public concerns. In an attempt to salvage the published research, a corrigendum was issued. Far from resolving the concerns raised, the corrigendum was itself criticized in anonymous PubPeer comments for containing further errors in October 2019.

For Better Science: A crowd-sourced project running a website with the help of an international team of research integrity experts.

Retraction Watch: A blog dedicated to reporting on research misconduct and tracking journal article retractions.

Following public criticism and online commentary, the University of Portsmouth convened a formal disciplinary panel in line with its procedure for the investigation of allegations of research misconduct in January 2020, according to the court records. While internal university reports are confidential, the 91-page 2024 high court judgment serves as the definitive public source of the investigation's evidence, the panel's conclusions, and the university's admission that the research failed to meet the required contractual standards of "reasonable skill and care." This legal ruling provides a comprehensive public record of the institutional investigation of the allegations of research misconduct. According to the court documents, the panel included independent external experts from other universities. The court judgment showed that the university's investigation panel concluded that misconduct in research had taken place. These findings were cited in the notice of the 2021 retraction of the 2019 *Cancer Letters* paper as the basis for retracting the paper. The retraction served as the catalyst for the subsequent breach of contract litigation, as the company sought to recover the loss resulting from the invalidated research.

In its court claim in 2023, the company alleged that the research misconduct at the University of Portsmouth, as confirmed in the 2020 investigation and reported in the 2021 retraction notice, had rendered its patent commercially worthless and necessitated the total repetition of the originally planned research program. The central allegations focused on whether the university had breached its 2016 research partnership agreement by failing to conduct research with integrity and whether the lead investigator had acted dishonestly or recklessly. The 2019 corrigendum served as part of the company's argument that, because even the corrected data were erroneous, the breach of contract was a systemic failure rather than a simple mistake. The judge found that the university was indeed in breach of contract. The court also examined allegations that the lead investigator had acted dishonestly or recklessly. The judge rejected the allegation of dishonesty and instead attributed the data errors to a "degree of carelessness" under professional pressure. The court ruled that the university's liability was capped by a specific clause in the research agreement, and the company was awarded £1 million in damages, the maximum amount permitted under the contractual limit.

In 2024, the university was ordered by the court to pay the company a £1 million settlement for breach of contract, following findings that the research failed to meet the contractual standard of "reasonable skill and care" (Box 8.2). The University of Portsmouth was ranked in the Shanghai Academic Ranking of World Universities in the 901–1000 band in 2025, fluctuating in different bands during the time period from 2017 onwards, when it was ranked 501–600. The pharmaceutical company was in liquidation at the time of writing this book (no causal inference is asserted or implied). Publicly available academic metrics for the lead researcher showed that he had an *h*-index of 34 according to Google Scholar in 2025. Since the 2021 retraction, he has had five papers included in the publications list and accrued over 200

Corrigendum: A correction notice concerning a paper's version of record when the error(s) in the research work do not impact the main findings.

Retraction: Removing a published paper from the research record due, for example, to the discovery of a flaw in its integrity.

Liquidation: The process of ending a business.

h(Hirsh)-index: A popular statistic to measure scientific output, taking account of citations, e.g., an *h*-index of 5 means that the author has 5 published papers that have been cited 5 times or more.

Journal quartiles: A journal metric based on citation performance (e.g., impact factor, CiteScore, etc.) ranking all journals in a field into four equal groups, Q1–Q4.

Google Scholar: A freely accessible web search engine that indexes scholarly literature across a wide range of formats and disciplines, aggregating nearly all major scholarly publishing.

citations per year. Publicly available blogs commenting on this case study also listed two additional retractions for papers on which he was a co-author (a 2011 Oncotarget paper retracted in 2019, and a 2017 Nature Communications paper retracted in 2023; DOIs: 10.18632/oncotarget.378; 10.1038/ncomms14687). The *Cancer Letters* journal impact factor was around 10, and it ranked in Q1 quartile in the cancer research category at the time of writing this book, having risen from an impact factor of around 7 (Q1 quartile) in 2019. According to the UK Charity Commission records, the charitable organizations involved did not see any drop in their annual income over the case study time period. Changes in institutional rankings, company status, charity income, academic indices, or journal metrics are reported descriptively only; no causal relationship with the case study is asserted or implied.

Box 8.2 Snapshot: The dimensions of research integrity issues in a case study of alleged breach of contract in Portsmouth

Actors and their research integrity roles (described without assessing their adequacy or compliance with standards)	**Reported observations over case study timeline** (no causal inference implied)
Institution: University of Portsmouth	
• Responsible for overseeing research conduct of its staff. • Responsible for investigating allegations of research misconduct under its published procedures. • Party with responsibility for research integrity in an academic-industry partnership established formally via a contract.	• Corrigendum and retraction of an article. • The finding of internal investigation became subject of examination in court. • Ordered to pay £1 million in compensation for breach of contract. • University's Shanghai ranking decreased.
Journal: *Cancer Letters* published by Elsevier	
• As the journal publishing the articles in question, it had responsibility to peer review the submitted manuscripts before publication. • Following post-publication peer review comments, it engaged promptly in corrections according to its publication integrity protocols.	• An October 2019 corrigendum followed by retraction in 2021 of a May 2019 article. • Journal impact factor increased and quartile ranking was unchanged.

Industry: A pharmaceutical company	
• Was a party in an academic-industry partnership established formally via a contract. • Funded the research conducted at the university.	• Awarded £1 million in compensation for breach of contract. • Entered liquidation proceedings following the conclusion of the litigation and the retraction of the associated research paper (no causal relationship between the litigation, retraction, and liquidation is asserted or implied).
Charitable sector	
• Two registered charitable organizations engaged in this work; one engaged direct in the academic-industry partnership agreement and the other underpinned the laboratory used for the research.	• According to the UK Charity Commission records, there was no drop in the income of the two registered charities.
Sleuthing	
• Sleuths made post-publication peer review comments on PubPeer. • Research integrity commentaries on blogs including For Better Science, Retraction Watch, and others.	• Data anomalies reported. • Blogs published covered the case on various research integrity outlets identifying further retractions.

See Box 1.1 for research integrity terminology.
See Box 1.2 for how research integrity concerns might arise and Box 1.3 for an outline of a research misconduct investigation.
See Box 8.1 for sources of information and the timeline of the case study.
Disclaimer: All factual statements are drawn from published literature and public records. No new allegation of research misconduct, dishonesty, or malice is intended or implied. The case study summarizes publicly available information and does not purport to determine liability or responsibility beyond what has been established in the cited records. References to individuals or organizations are made for academic discussion only and do not attribute intent or fault beyond the public record. When reporting changes in individual, institutional, organizational, and journal status or metrics, no causal inference is implied. The commentary and any opinions expressed are offered in good faith on matters of public interest concerning research integrity. Readers are encouraged to consult the original sources for full context.
University ranking data source: URL: www.shanghairanking.com/rankings/arwu/#### (year).
Journal impact factor and ranking are based on Journal Citation Reports.
Charitable organization data obtained from URL: register-of-charities.charitycommission.gov.uk.

Research integrity concerns for charities

Drawing from the court judgment, retraction notice, and public records summarized above, the following analysis examines the vulnerabilities charities face in funding research and offers recommendations for strengthening oversight.

While medical research charities are a pivotal third pillar of funders, they are often uniquely vulnerable to research misconduct, as they may operate without the stringent oversight frameworks utilized by government or large commercial funders. This case discusses vulnerabilities that may arise in the oversight of charity-funded research. It sheds light on how charities can engage in academic research with universities. The charities were formally named in the acknowledgment section of the published *Cancer Letters* paper. There were numerous public criticisms. A corrigendum, which was subsequently criticized on post-publication peer review platforms as containing errors, was issued, and then the paper was retracted following a finding of misconduct in research as stated in the retraction notice. The court judgment examined findings from the university investigation concerning failures to meet contractual research integrity standards. This type of outcome directly poses reputational risk to the charities. They might, with hindsight, even wonder how they came to be embroiled in research and publication integrity failures despite all their good intentions.

Transparency in research: Open research practices including prospective registration, adherence to study design, *a priori* statistical analysis plan, data sharing, timely and complete public reporting, conflict of interest disclosure, open research assessment, open publication practice, etc.

Funding effect: The pressure to prove a specific hypothesis linked to a secondary interest (financial or contractual) associated with funding.

Best-practice frameworks emphasize that reliance on institutional oversight alone, without independent verification, may increase risk exposure for charities. Research integrity requires undertaking research according to strict ethical and professional standards. However, when charities fund research institutions, the responsibility to oversee research conduct is assumed by the awardee. Institutional due diligence requires a clear and published procedure for investigating allegations of research misconduct that can withstand legal scrutiny. If the pressure to produce positive findings for fundraising campaigns inadvertently incentivizes a deviation from the standards, then the risk to research integrity becomes high. Charities should move beyond the fund and hope for the best model toward active due diligence (Box 8.3). Mandatory institutional confirmation that staff have no outstanding sanctions for research misconduct, independent third-party audits of raw data, a requirement for immediate notification on commencing formal investigations, the right to sanction both individuals and institutions, and clawback rights in cases of breach of contract through research misconduct are all necessary steps for charities to protect their mission and reputation.

Box 8.3 Medical research charities: Suggestions for managing research integrity risks

Due diligence feature	Comments
Pre-award diligence	Require universities to confirm that the applicants submitting a grant application have no outstanding sanctions or active investigations for misconduct. Failure of disclosure may warrant organizational sanctions, subject to applicable policies and due process.
Grant peer review	Integrity of work leading to the proposals should be assessed formally, e.g., examining for retracted citations or expressions of concern in the bibliography as well as comments and responses on public post-publication peer review platforms. Experts including individuals with relevant knowledge or experience in a given subject area such as academic researchers, clinicians, industry representatives, and regulators, as well as patients, people with lived experience, service users, and other interested members of the public should provide independent advice to the research review committee drawn from a pool of experts.
Institutional research governance	Confirm that the host institution has a culture that reinforces integrity with robust research governance, and regular internal audit processes for oversight. Complete and accurate research documentation is the primary proof of due diligence.
Independent verification	Implement independent, third-party audits or inspections of studies they fund; reliance solely on institutional internal oversight is insufficient.
Research integrity standards and charity-led investigations	Verify that the host institution has publicly documented research integrity policies and procedures before funding. Institutions must inform the charity immediately upon a decision to formally investigate an allegation of research misconduct against a funded researcher. Charities should reserve the right to suspend or terminate a grant if an act of research misconduct or questionable practice adversely affects the charity's name or reputation. Charities should reserve the right to observe research misconduct inquiry panels or undertake their own investigations depending on the circumstances. They may apply sanctions against entire institutions if they fail to investigate integrity concerns promptly and objectively. Investigation reports serve as primary evidence in breach of contract cases. Sanctions may include letters of reprimand, restriction from future funding, and repayment of the grant.

Funding disclosures	All publications must have transparent funding disclosures, mentioning the charitable organization contribution in a manner this is explicit.
Data integrity and preservation	Mandate that raw data must be retained for a specified time period and specifically require original, unmanipulated image files to be preserved alongside processed versions. Every data item and graph must be treated as a legal representation of the research project.
Transparency, data shraring, and openness	Ensure that institutions funded have policies in practice for reporting of suspected misconduct in a responsible and appropriate manner. In some jurisdictions, the regulators of charities require reporting of serious incidents such as research misconduct by a partner. Protocols, registrations, preprints, and final manuscripts must be publicly accessible, supporting open science with data sharing. Public has a right to expect the integrity of charity-funded research and report concerns.
Conflict management	Charities must publish a conflicts of interest policy for their funding awards. Policies must ensure research is free from bias involving a funded researcher's financial and non-financial interests. Researchers engaged in charity-funded research projects should not be placed under pressure to produce positive findings, prioritizing integrity and quality. Both honest errors and deliberate misconduct can undermine trust.
Publication integrity standards	Publishing with integrity is a contractual duty for institutions. Charities should actively monitor post-publication peer review comments and must be vigilant about rapid fixes (corrigenda) by researchers when underlying data are challenged in their funded projects. Persistent errors in a corrigendum can be evidence systemic failure. Charities may require the formal retraction or republication with correction of published papers produced by researchers funded by them.

Source: URLs: wellcome.org/research-funding/guidance/policies-grant-conditions/responsible-conduct-research; www.bhf.org.uk/for-professionals/information-for-researchers/how-to-apply/standard-conditions-of-grants; www.amrc.org.uk/research-guidance.

Chapter 8: Alleged misconduct in charity-funded research: Breach of contract and an investigation in Portsmouth – Key points

Advice for researchers

- Beware that failure to meet contractual research integrity standards may give rise to breach-of-contract liability in court.
- Researchers must treat every data item and graph as a legal representation of their work.
- Documentation is due diligence. Integrity is proven through a clear audit trail. Poor record-keeping can be interpreted as a failure to exercise reasonable skill and care.
- The post-publication lifespan can be short or long. Integrity issues can surface any time after a project ends. Researchers remain professionally liable for the integrity of their data.
- Engage in whistleblowing when necessary. If research and publication misconduct or questionable practices are suspected, report promptly in writing to relevant bodies, e.g., funders or journals.

Recommendations for journals and publishers

- Integrate image-forensic tools into due diligence process during submission, editorial assessment, and peer review, not just after a complaint is made (see Chapter 7).
- Be vigilant about the corrigendum trap. Permitting rapid fixes (corrigenda) when the underlying integrity of the data is challenged is risky.
- Fast-tracked integrity investigations with the input of institutions are key (Box 1.3); journals have a duty to act rapidly to avoid misleading the public or other researchers.
- When concerns arise about published research that has received funding, notify the funders promptly to enable coordinated responses and to limit downstream reputational and legal risks.

Roles of institutions and funders

- Institutions must implement rigorous research governance with internal audits to ensure their researchers' work doesn't expose them to legal risks (see Box 10.3 for an institutional action plan).
- Investment in a research integrity culture with mandatory training and updates is a must as institutions are liable for their employees' work.

COPE: Committee on Publication Ethics issues guidance to journals on responsible publication practices, including handling research misconduct allegations.

ICMJE: International Committee of Medical Journal Editors provides guidance to journals on publishing policies, such as public prospective registration, data sharing, conflict of interest declaration, authorship criteria, etc.

WAME: World Association of Medical Editors. It aims to improve editorial standards through self-regulation.

- Institutional due diligence requires a clear, published procedure for investigating allegations of misconduct (Box 1.3), as these findings serve as evidence in court.
- Funders, including both industry and charities, should have independent data verification through an independent, third-party audit or inspection of the raw data instead of reliance solely on institutional internal oversight. Major public or fundraising campaigns demand this level of scrutiny.
- Before signing research partnership agreements, industry and charity partners must assess the research integrity record as part of the due diligence process. Charities must consider reputational risk as a factor in their due diligence, ensuring they have an exit strategy if research misconduct is uncovered.
- Funders should include clawback rights in research agreements, allowing recovery of funds in cases where research misconduct or breach of contract is established (Box 8.3).

Research culture: The academic environment comprising the norms, values, expectations, attitudes, and behaviors within research organizations. Academic freedom, collegiality, collaboration, equality and diversity, research integrity (ethics and professionalism), conflict management with openness, accountability, and transparency are all features of the research culture.

9 *Authorial credit and accountability*

Retraction and reported guest authorship in Amsterdam

All authors taking credit for an article are meant to take responsibility for the work they publish. The case study in this chapter centers on a 2011 clinical study published in the *Gynecological Endocrinology* journal, retracted in 2024 over alleged data integrity concerns, after which additional authorship issues were publicly disclosed. A co-author from the University of Amsterdam confessed in a journal article she wrote that her inclusion as an author was guest authorship, an honorary gift, for which she made no substantive contribution. This sequence of events reframed the retraction as a case in point for discussing questionable authorship practices and the associated research culture. The analysis explores the systemic drivers of guest authorship, its kinship with falsification and plagiarism, and the severe personal and professional repercussions for those involved. Crucially, it highlights the principle of collective authorial responsibility, arguing that all named authors share accountability for a paper's integrity, regardless of their individual roles. The chapter will conclude that retractions, while correcting the scientific record, can also serve as powerful tools for exposing and reforming the opaque norms of authorship attribution, advocating for strict adherence to established authorship criteria to preserve trust in scholarly communication.

Research integrity: Undertaking research and publication following ethical and professional principles and standards. Responsible research and publication practices pave the way for science to be regarded as trustworthy. Integrity failures may result from honest errors or deliberate misconduct.

Asymmetry of credit and accountability in guest authorship

Academia is competitive, with the term publish or perish being its recognized survival guide. Authorship is the formal attribution of credit to individuals who have made a substantial intellectual contribution to a scholarly work, conferring both recognition for the effort and accountability for the work's integrity. Thus, in the academic profession, authorship is one of the primary currencies of prestige; the other being citations (see Chapter 2). It is the definitive metric used for hiring, promotion, grant funding, and professional status in the world of academia. Authorship contains a dual role. The reward for intellectual labor versus the pledge of responsibility creates a powerful tension. Notably, when the pressure to accumulate publications

Publish or perish: An academic culture in which institutions value the number of papers rather than their quality or their impact.

DOI: 10.1201/9781003655916-9

incentivizes research misconduct, such as guest authorship, it undermines the integrity of the very system of academic evaluation it is meant to underpin.

A central contradiction in guest authorship is the selective embrace of academic capital. Gift, courtesy, and honorary authorship are other synonyms for the same concept. Some researchers have acknowledged accepting authorship without substantive contribution, incorporating the unearned publication into their CVs, promotion dossiers, and grant applications. This credit is actively leveraged for professional advancement, reinforcing a system where perceived productivity, rather than genuine intellectual contribution, is rewarded. For example, a proportion of highly prolific authors (those publishing one paper every five days or more than 72 full papers annually) have reportedly admitted failing to meet authorship criteria (DOI: 10.1038/d41586-018-06185-8). The guest author benefits from the prestige that comes with high publication numbers and any resulting citations. There is institutional recognition that the publications and the associated citations indicate esteem; however, all this is achieved without having invested any or minimal effort in the studies' conception, execution, or validation. This practice can have the effect of treating authorship as a form of academic currency, which, when detached from scholarly labor, risks diminishing its meaning as a marker of genuine intellectual contribution and responsibility. Guest authorship has been described by some research integrity scholars as research misconduct in that it aligns with falsification, as credit is not accurately represented in the research record (DOI: 10.1136/bmjebm-2021-111826). Moreover, the same source noted that guest authorship could also align with plagiarism, i.e., authors claim to have substantially contributed when, in fact, they have only appropriated or claimed a portion of credit for the work reported by the actual authors. These reported arguments imply that guest authorship can be said to meet two of the three cardinal integrity sins enshrined in the classical research misconduct definition, abbreviated as FFP (fabrication, falsification, plagiarism), even if it is not formally classified as such.

The calculus of the dual role of authorship, combining credit and responsibility, can dramatically reverse when the foundational integrity of the work, co-authored via guest authorship, collapses publicly. Upon retraction, prompted by reported data integrity concerns and other issues identified during post-publication peer review, the very same individuals who originally accepted guest authorship may seek to distance themselves from responsibility following a retraction. They retreat behind claims of ignorance (Box 9.1), minor contribution, or lack of oversight (Chapter 4), attempting to frame their involvement

Authorship abuse: Unethical authorship, naming authors not strictly based on contribution, e.g., guest authorship.

Guest authorship: Listing as co-authors those who have not made substantial contributions. Synonyms of guest include gift, courtesy, honorary, etc.

Accountability: A responsible research principle guiding individuals and organizations to be answerable for the research they engage in from idea to post-publication.

Institution: An academic organization, typically a university, where research takes place. It has the responsibility to oversee ethical and professional research conduct.

Plagiarism: Copying the work of others (text, tables, images, data, etc.) and presenting it as one's own work without proper citation to the source.

FFP: Fabrication, falsification, and plagiarism.

as non-substantive or peripheral. This stance directly contradicts the foundational principle of collective accountability for all authors upheld by leading research and publication integrity bodies, including the European Code of Conduct for Research Integrity (URL: allea.org/code-of-conduct) and the International Committee of Medical Journal Editors (ICMJE) (URL: www.icmje.org/icmje-recommendations.pdf). As exemplified by some published decisions of the Swedish National Board for Assessment of Research Misconduct, all authors share responsibility for the content of the publication unless otherwise stated (URL: npof.se/en/decisions; cases 3.1-22-0191 and 3.2-22-0092). As the rules and the cases underscore, established research integrity frameworks emphasize that authorship entails both credit and shared responsibility, such that authors cannot fully disclaim accountability for a publication's integrity once concerns emerge, even if their role was limited. This discrepancy between credit and responsibility illustrates how guest authorship can undermine established principles of scholarly accountability and may erode confidence in academic authorship practices. It corrupts the incentive structure of academia, allowing individuals to profit from a system they simultaneously fail to uphold, ultimately demanding that authorship be re-anchored to tangible contribution and unwavering accountability. This chapter explores a case study of a retraction for alleged data integrity concerns in which additional authorship issues were publicly disclosed.

Retraction: Removing a published paper from the research record due, for example, to the discovery of a flaw in its integrity.

ICMJE: International Committee of Medical Journal Editors provides guidance to journals on publishing policies, such as public prospective registration, data sharing, conflict of interest declaration, authorship criteria, etc.

PubPeer: An online platform for post-publication peer review.

Box 9.1 Retraction watch: "Sleuth loses paper for duplicate publication" claiming "was not aware"

Background

- A 2016–17 clinical trial with an authorship representing a Global North–South research partnership involving Australia and Vietnam was published in the journal *Obstetrics & Gynecology* in March 2019, with the developed country partner appearing as last author in senior position.
- The paper was submitted, peer reviewed, revised, and accepted in October–December 2018. The published article stated: "Each author has confirmed compliance with the journal's requirements for authorship."
- The paper also stated that the work had been presented at various professional society meetings in the US and Singapore earlier in 2018 but made no mention of any other prior publication.

Retraction

- In 2025, the 2019 *Obstetrics & Gynecology* paper was retracted for being a duplicate publication, with the same authorship. Before retraction it had already been cited around 60 times according to Google Scholar.
- Originally, it had been published the *Vietnamese Journal of Obstetrics and Gynecology* in May 2018, where it was submitted, revised, and accepted in April 2018.
- The original journals' publication system required an explicit signed statement that "all authors contributed to the research, prepared the manuscript, and are jointly responsible for the content of the manuscript" (translated from Vietnamese document on journal website).

Post-retraction comment

- Retraction Watch blog, interviewing the Australian author from Monash University, reported that he "was not aware" of the original Vietnamese publication.
- The blog also explained how the retracted senior author claiming ignorance had been a sleuth himself.
- A comment on the Retraction Watch blog stated that "any reasonable person would not accept the claim that a senior author is unaware of two publications. In such a case, he would be accepting guest authorship, and all his publications would need to be scrutinized."
- The 2018 article was listed on the senior author's publication list on his Google Scholar and ResearchGate profiles making it discoverable as the original alongside the 2019 duplicate publication.

See Box 9.4 for some recommendations for authorship integrity in Global North–South research collaborations.
See Box 7.1 for accountability as a research integrity principle.
This box summarizes reported allegations and findings in the sources listed below; no judgment is intended.
Sources: DOIs: 10.46755/vjog.2018.1.693; 10.1097/AOG.0000000000003136; 10.1097/AOG.0000000000006043. URLs: vjog.vn/journal/about/submissions; retractionwatch.com/2025/10/15/sleuth-loses-paper-for-duplicate-publication-after-flagging-hundreds-of-untrustworthy-articles; pubpeer.com/publications/F006A3F6D238BEA427E0B26F60BD4A; www.facebook.com/share/p/1CDg1HoATc; scholar.google.com/citations?view_op=view_citation&hl=es&user=900W_JMAAAAJ&cstart=1000&pagesize=100&sortby=pubdate&citation_for_view=900W_JMAAAAJ%3A8bEfNjzhQ0EC; https://www.researchgate.net/publication/343529431_Vong_nang_co_tu_cung_so_voi_progesterone_dat_am_dao_trong_phong_ngua_sinh_non_o_thai_phu_mang_song_thai_co_chieu_dai_co_tu_cung_38_mm_mot_thu_nghiem_ngau_nhien_co_nhom_chung.

A case study of guest authorship

This case study summarizes information from publicly available PubPeer comments, a retraction notice, and peer-reviewed publications, and discusses them in the context of research integrity scholarship.

In an international multicountry collaboration involving the Netherlands and Egypt, a study conducted from 2004 to 2008 was

Shanghai ranking: Academic Ranking of World Universities, one of the most influential global research-based university rankings.

published in 2011, co-authored by researchers affiliated with institutions in both countries. At the time of publication, the University of Amsterdam, one of the affiliated institutions, ranked 101–150 in the Shanghai Academic Ranking of World Universities. The study was published as an article in *Gynecological Endocrinology* (Box 9.2), the official journal of the International Society of Gynecological Endocrinology, a non-profit organization for promoting research into all aspects of gynecological endocrinology. The journal publisher was Taylor & Francis, a leading global academic publisher with around 2700 academic journals across diverse fields, including the humanities, social sciences, and medicine. The journal impact factor was less than 2, and it ranked in Q3 among journals in the obstetrics and gynecology category in 2011.

Impact factor: A journal statistic dividing the mean number of citations per article in a year by the total number of citable articles published in the previous two years.

The retraction notice stated that the retraction was made by the editor and publisher, and it cited both the failure to verify data integrity due to the unavailability of data, owing to the study's age, and concerns over authorship qualifications, explicitly linking the two issues. Until this point, the guest authorship arrangement, an informal practice justified as professional courtesy, had remained undisclosed. The case study paper itself lacked any contributorship statement. Post-retraction commentary raised concerns about this issue as one of the University of Amsterdam authors stated in a 2024 commentary published in the *Fertility and Sterility* journal (DOI: 10.1016/j.fertnstert.2023.10.005) that she "had not even read the manuscript" prior to publication, reflecting on her involvement. The admission originally occurred in her own article published online before the formal retraction, which may indicate that the disclosure was linked to the publisher's investigation, which stated in the retraction notice that the journal was "also made aware of concerns regarding whether all the authors listed in the publication qualify for authorship according to the journal's editorial policies." As the implicated guest author came forward with this admission publicly, this transformed the case from a statistical correction into a stark, personal narrative of research misattribution. During the 10+ years following publication, the article and its associated citations would have been available in her record, contributing to her professional stature.

Journal quartiles: A journal metric based on citation performance (e.g., impact factor, CiteScore, etc.) ranking all journals in a field into four equal groups, Q1–Q4.

Box 9.2 Timeline of research integrity concerns: A case study of retraction and reported gift authorship in Amsterdam

Dates	Brief overview of events
2010–11	**Article submission, peer review, and publication** The paper was submitted in 2010 and accepted following peer review. The study had reportedly been conducted 2004–2008 after obtaining human research ethics committee approval. It was published in 2011. There were two named authors from the University of Amsterdam. The paper's conflict of interest declaration stated that the "authors alone are responsible for the content and writing of the paper." A note of correction stated that an author had been missed from the author list, but this was an Egyptian not an Amsterdam author. There was no contributorship statement providing the role(s) for individual authors. *Source: DOI: 10.3109/09513590.2010.540600.*
November 2023	**Post-publication peer review** PubPeer comments identified data integrity issues. *Sources: URL: pubpeer.com/publications/C86E576602BB28E AE06786CAC278B3.*
February 2024	**Authorship misconduct commentary article** One of the Amsterdam authors of the 2011 paper wrote in a commentary article that she had been added to the authorship of the article because the co-author told her that "people in his country would be nowhere without friends helping other friends further in life. I pleaded him not to use my name like this anymore, and that was it. I decided not to retract my name, although I had not even read the manuscript." She further explained that in "guest authorship, also known as gift or honorary authorship, people are made coauthors although they did not really contribute to the manuscript ... Guest authorship can also be used to repay a favor or maintain good relationships with colleagues and collaboration partners." The quotation is reproduced verbatim from the published source and is presented for analytical purposes, without endorsement or generalization beyond the individual account. The publication date of this commentary article (published online October 2023) and that of the PubPeer comments about data integrity (published November 2023) appear discrepant. *Sources: DOI: 10.1016/j.fertnstert.2023.10.005.*

September 2024	**Retraction** The journal stated that it followed COPE guidelines. The retraction notice stated that the journal was "also made aware of concerns regarding whether all the authors listed in the publication qualify for authorship according to the journal's editorial policies." *Source: DOI: 10.1080/09513590.2024.2401196.*
September 2024	**Guest authorship** One of the Amsterdam authors wrote on PubPeer: "Though it has been a difficult decision for the authors involved, it is good that this paper has now been retracted. Sadly enough I had a guest authorship on this paper (https://www.fertstert.org/article/S0015-0282(23)01920-9/fulltext)" referring to the authorship misconduct commentary article. A response to this post said, "It is essential to recognize that the guest author still benefited by obtaining credit from the work that others have done and including the 'unearned' publication on their resume as evidence of academic productivity. How is this any different than one using a non-existing article as a proof of productivity and not correcting the error even when made aware?" Another response asked the Amsterdam author, "Do you believe it is appropriate to continue holding positions on the editorial boards of journals under these circumstances?" There was no reply. *Source: URL: pubpeer.com/publications/C86E576602BB28EAE06786CAC278B3.*

See Box 9.3 for an outline of the research integrity roles of various actors in this case study, along with the disclaimer.
Sources listed above are a few of the many that have covered this case study. This box summarizes reported allegations and findings; no judgment is intended.

This case study has been discussed as illustrative of challenges that can arise in some Global North–South research collaborations. It lays bare entrenched practices, exploring how authorship abuses are systematically enabled and justified, and are only rarely challenged. The insight gained connects the micro-ethics of authorship criteria to the macro-ethics of global knowledge production, highlighting that true research decolonization requires not only equitable data sharing and funding but also radical transparency and fairness in the attribution of authorship credit. At the time of writing, the author who publicly reported having held guest authorship remained employed at the institution. Publicly available bibliometric indicators on Google

h(Hirsh)-index: A popular statistic to measure scientific output, taking account of citations, e.g., an *h*-index of 5 means that the author has 5 published papers that have been cited 5 times or more.

Scholar listed her *h*-index as 75 in 2025. The paper in question had been cited around 120 times in total before retraction, according to Google Scholar. The University of Amsterdam maintained its ranking within the 101–150 band in the Shanghai Academic Ranking of World Universities in 2025 (Box 9.3). The recent *Gynecological Endocrinology* journal impact factor was under 2, and it ranked in Q2 among journals in the category of obstetrics and gynecology, whereas it had been ranked lower in Q3 in 2011. Changes in institutional rankings, article-level citations, academic indices, or journal metrics are reported descriptively only; no causal relationship with the case study is asserted or implied.

Google Scholar: A freely accessible web search engine that indexes scholarly literature across a wide range of formats and disciplines, aggregating nearly all major scholarly publishing.

Box 9.3 Snapshot: The dimensions of research integrity issues in a case study of retraction and reported gift authorship in Amsterdam

Actors and their research integrity roles (described without assessing adequacy or compliance with standards)	**Reported observations over case study timeline** (no causal inference implied)
Institution: University of Amsterdam	
• Responsible for overseeing research conduct of its staff. • Responsible for investigating allegations of research misconduct under its policies and procedures.	• Retracted article. • Staff identified in published commentary as having held guest authorship. • Related authorship integrity commentary published in a peer-reviewed journal. • No public record of an institutional investigation found; such an internal inquiry may not have beeen made public. • University's Shanghai ranking unchanged.
Journal: *Gynecological Endocrinology*, the official journal of the International Society of Gynecological Endocrinology and published by Taylor & Francis	

• Responsible for editorial assessment and peer review of the submitted manuscripts before publication. • Responsible for timely investigation of post-publication integrity concerns raised under journal editorial policies supported by the publisher's research integrity team.	• A 2011 article retracted in 2024 after journal investigation. • The journal impact factor and quartile ranking increased.
Sleuthing	
• Sleuths made post-publication and post-retraction comments on PubPeer.	• Post-publication comments identified data integrity concerns in 2023. • Post-retraction comments on the guest authorship admission in 2024.

See Box 1.1 for research integrity terminology.
See Box 1.2 for how research integrity concerns might arise and Box 1.3 for an outline of a research misconduct investigation.
See Box 9.2 for sources of information and the timeline of the case study.
Disclaimer: All factual statements are drawn from published literature and public records. No new allegation of research misconduct, dishonesty, or malice is intended or implied. The case study summarizes publicly available information and does not purport to determine liability or responsibility beyond what has been established in the cited records. References to individuals or organizations are made for academic discussion only and do not attribute intent or fault beyond the public record. When reporting changes in individual, institutional, organizational, and journal status or metrics, no causal inference is implied. The commentary and any opinions expressed are offered in good faith on matters of public interest concerning research integrity. Readers are encouraged to consult the original sources for full context.
University ranking data source: URL: www.shanghairanking.com/rankings/arwu/#### (year).
Journal impact factor and ranking are based on Journal Citation Reports.

Ethics dumping: Decolonizing authorship

Ethics dumping: Exploitative practices, taking advantage of the imbalance of power, in research partnerships between high-, middle-, and low-income settings.

The case study above provides an entry point for examining broader systemic issues in Global North–South research collaborations. The following analysis, drawing on the case and the cited literature, explores how authorship practices can reflect and reinforce power imbalances.

This phenomenon of guest authorship has been examined through the revelatory lens of an article retraction in this case. However, the issue of authorship integrity is fraught with complexities, in part because of the controversy surrounding the recommended criteria and in part because of the way power is exercised in academic corridors to bend them. Some commentators have argued that the ICMJE authorship criteria may be insufficiently flexible across diverse disciplinary and cultural contexts. The pressure to publish within the academic publish or perish culture fosters widespread abuse, including guest authorship, where credit is detached from genuine contribution. In this broader context, the risk of inequitable credit allocation in collaborations with low–middle-income country co-authors is a phenomenon that warrants specific attention. Ethics dumping and parachute research are related terms. This case study of a retraction exposing guest authorship serves as an entry point for discussion about the complex and often exploitative dynamics of Global North–South research collaborations. Beyond a simple breach of publication norms, this case illuminates how authorship can be commodified, gifted, or exploited within partnerships marked by inherent power imbalances.

The ethical imperative to include colleague researchers from low-resource settings as legitimate co-authors requires moving beyond paternalistic colonial traditions. The integrity of scientific authorship, a fundamental pillar of research integrity, cannot remain unevenly distributed across the global academic landscape. In many such collaborations, researchers from institutions in the Global North and South engage in joint projects where resources, prestige, and influence tend to be asymmetrical. A breach of authorship integrity in this context is the practice of guest authorship, where researchers from Northern institutions are listed as authors on work undertaken by Southern teams without substantive contribution, often to lend credibility or facilitate publication in journals. These practices extend beyond administrative concerns and have been discussed in the literature as contributing to inequities in authorship credit. They reinforce historic colonial hierarchies where Northern names carry symbolic capital, while the substantial, on-the-ground research contributions of Southern scholars are undervalued or obscured. Ultimately, the responsibility lies with institutions, funders, and journals to reform the culture and structures, enforce ethical and professional standards, and protect the integrity of the authorship process, ensuring that credit accurately reflects the collective effort in multicountry research partnerships. Whenever there is a power imbalance, the responsibility for avoiding abuse in the asymmetrical relationship lies with the powerful, not the weak.

This case study underscores that until authorship is decoupled from power and realigned with contribution, the scholarly record will remain a contested site of visibility and privilege. Empirical evidence of authorship inequity shows that low–middle-income country authors are underrepresented in Global North–South collaborations, missing completely from authorship and named infrequently in first and corresponding author roles (DOIs: 10.1093/ije/dyw313; 10.2991/

Parachute research: Exploitative practice where researchers from high-income settings collect data and samples from lower-income settings, without local involvement or collaboration.

Colonization of research: A systemic mindset and power structure that perpetuates historical colonial hierarchies in Global North–South research partnerships.

Power: Abuse of role asymmetry. In Global North–South research collaborations, researchers from institutions in developed countries enjoy more resources, prestige, and influence compared to their less developed country partners, opening the door to the possibility of authorship abuse.

jegh.k.200325.001). This case study provides an example of another type of abuse pertaining not to the exclusion of low–middle-income country authors, but to the inappropriate inclusion of high-income country collaborators via guest authorship. This way, high-income country guest authorship in the works of low–middle-income countries may be criticized as a colonial patronage practice, reinforcing power imbalances, to seek legitimization of the work for publication in journals where editors and peer reviewers tend to come from high-income countries. Key solutions include employing detailed contributorship statements, using systems like CRediT (DOI: 10.21037/atm.2019.12.96), to explicitly document each individual author's role(s). The persistent authorship inequities demand more than passive guidelines; they require proactive, structural reforms that address the power imbalances at the heart of North–South collaborations (Box 9.4). The paradigm needs to shift from voluntary compliance to enforceable accountability, ensuring that authorship credit is aligned with genuine intellectual labor and that research partnerships become truly reciprocal. By embedding equitable authorship into institutional policies and funding agreements, the responsibility for ethical practice will be transferred from the individual researcher to the institution and the partnership structure itself. These lessons provide a foundation for the practical guidance that follows in the key points section.

CRediT: Contributor Roles Taxonomy is a system for classifying the roles played by individual authors and those acknowledged in a scholarly publication.

Box 9.4 Some recommendations for authorship integrity in research collaborations beyond borders

Feature	Comments
Transparent contribution	Mandate detailed individual contributorship statements specifying each author's individual role(s) to increase accountability instead of bundling authorship into ICMJE combined criteria. Authorship criteria have been criticized as insufficiently adaptable in some contexts as they can be systematically biased against low- and middle-income setting unless substantial efforts are made, e.g., counting critical review of translated drafts as intellectual contribution. To avoid post-hoc conflicts and manage expectations, authorship agreements should be developed at the start and kept under review for contributions and order.
Authorship order	Address power issues via clear, agreed-upon criteria for authorship order to avoid automatic assignment of prestige positions such as first, last, and corresponding authorships. Use joint authorship at prestige positions to share credit equitably.

Open science	Require data sharing and joint data ownership to prevent parachute research that exploits power to exercise intellectual control on publication opportunities.
Editorial practices	Journals should reduce bias toward powerful authors and actively avoid perpetuating authorship inequities by monitoring for potential authorship irregularities. Diversifying editorial boards, editors, and peer reviewers will be a step in the right direction.
Institutional and funding stance	Institutions and funders should provide training in authorship ethics focusing on power dynamics, cultural differences, and fair credit allocation. Empower vulnerable researchers (e.g., early career or those from low- and middle-income setting) to negotiate authorship fairly and recognize unethical practices like guest authorship.
Recognize responsibility	In asymmetric relationships, the responsibility for avoiding abuse always lies with the powerful partner, not the vulnerable. Avoid shifting blame to co-authors from low- and middleincome country settings in cases of high-income country authorship concerns such as guest authorship.
Consequence acceptance	Claiming ignorance, shifting blame, and seeking forgiveness in the form of an apology post-retraction is not a substitute for authorship accountability (see Box 9.1). Demonstrate willingness to accept responsibility for possible failures to uphold authorship integrity standards.
Equitable partnership declaration	Journals should judiciously seek declarations from author groups to ensure that the contributions made by the researchers, academics, clinicians, communities, and other contributors based in the locations or sites of the research are described. These should be published with the papers.

See Box 7.1 for accountability as a research integrity principle.
Sources: DOIs: 10.1016/S2214-109X(23)00278-4; 10.1111/anae.15597; 10.1201/9781003461401; 10.21037/atm.2019.12.96. URL: wame.org/promoting-global-health.

Chapter 9: Authorial credit and accountability: Retraction and reported guest authorship in Amsterdam – Key points

Advice for researchers

- Credit and responsibility are inseparable in authorship as part of professional accountability (Box 7.1).
- Guest authorship is widely regarded as a high-risk practice and is treated by many research integrity frameworks as a serious breach of authorship standards amounting to misconduct.
- Vigilance is a core duty in authorship requiring integrity of one's own contributions and trust in collaborators. A lack of awareness or failure to scrutinize co-authors' work is not a valid defense when integrity failures become public.
- Deviation from authorship criteria, even for perceived cultural or collegial reasons, invites misconduct allegations.
- In asymmetric research partnerships, the responsibility for avoiding abuse lies with the powerful, not the vulnerable (Box 9.4). Transferring blame to the vulnerable is a failure of accountability.

Recommendations for journals and publishers

- Publishers should establish centralized research integrity teams as an industry standard and a core professionalized publishing function. This team should provide the expertise needed by editors to investigate cases when integrity concerns are raised (Box 1.3).
- Journals must implement and enforce robust verification, including confirming contributions, e.g., using CRediT taxonomy (DOI: 10.21037/atm.2019.12.96), with all listed authors and questioning the inclusion of individuals in purely prestige roles.
- Retractions may draw attention to broader ethical and professional issues, e.g., uncovering breaches like authorship misconduct in addition to data integrity issues. Journals must be prepared to engage in scrutinizing all allegations that emerge in investigations.
- Post-publication scrutiny on academic platforms outside journal-based correspondence and letters is a critical corrective tool for the scientific community to self-correct. Journals should have clear pathways to engage with concerns raised post-publication and treat them as integral to safeguarding the record, particularly where there is a lack of institutional investigations.

Roles of institutions and funders

- Organizational incentives drive behavior. Authorship integrity cannot be implemented without reforming the publish or perish culture (see Chapter 10 for institutional research culture).
- Hold all authors collectively responsible for research integrity. Incorporate authorship accountability in research integrity training (Box 7.1).
- Power imbalances enable exploitation of senior–junior collaborations, leading to guest authorship. Institutions should play an active role in preventing authorship abuse.
- In Global North–South research collaborations, power dynamics can lead to guest authorship (adding prestigious names from high-income country institutions). Institutions and funders must develop and enforce policies that mandate equitable authorship, recognizing that the responsibility for avoiding abuse lies with the powerful partners. Systemic reform is required for dismantling exploitative authorship practices rooted in historical inequities.

10 *Institutional research culture*

Alleged ethical failure and patient harm in Stockholm

Ethical integrity, the commitment to conduct research in accordance with moral principles and standards, demands that human research proceed only with a rigorous ethics review and fully informed consent. A landmark 2011 publication in *The Lancet* presented a proof-of-concept study involving a case report of a single patient, the lowest form of evidence in the evidence-based medicine hierarchy. The study was multi-authored, had funding from many prominent funders, and involved a multicountry, multidisciplinary collaboration of institutions led by the Swedish Karolinska Institute, which is renowned for organizing the Nobel Prize for physiology or medicine. However, by 2014, whistleblower concerns emerged, raising doubts about ethical approval, consent, data accuracy, and patient outcomes. External and internal institutional investigations in 2015 yielded conflicting results, with an initial misconduct finding overturned, but a 2016 television documentary and further probes revealed discrepancies in reporting, ethical approval, and consent processes. An expression of concern was issued in 2016, as some original co-authors asked for their names to be removed from the paper. A definitive external investigation confirmed deviations from responsible research practices, as documented in the findings of the publicly available report. *The Lancet* paper was retracted in 2018 amid findings of misconduct reported in investigations, alongside several other retractions of articles by the lead researcher. There were subsequent reforms in research oversight, including the establishment of the Swedish national research misconduct board. The case culminated in a 2023 court ruling giving a prison sentence to the lead researcher. This chapter will serve as a cautionary tale on balancing innovation with scientific integrity in biomedical research.

Research integrity: Undertaking research and publication following ethical and professional principles and standards. Responsible research and publication practices pave the way for science to be regarded as trustworthy. Integrity failures may result from honest errors or deliberate misconduct.

Institution: An academic organization, typically a university, where research takes place. It has the responsibility to oversee ethical and professional research conduct.

Ethics: Decision-making based on moral values that distinguish between right and wrong.

Ethical integrity in research and publication

From the lessons of Nuremberg and Helsinki, one might reasonably expect that in the 21st century, in a Northern European country that is the custodian of the Nobel Prize for medicine and renowned for

DOI: 10.1201/9781003655916-10

high ethical standards, no experimental procedure in human research would proceed without rigorous ethics review and fully informed consent. Ethics is the first of the two pillars of research integrity; the second is professionalism. The ethical principles and standards directly lead researchers to seek human research ethics committee approval and informed consent. Institutions have a responsibility to establish research ethics committees for approval and research governance offices, as mandated by law. This committee is different from hospitals' ethics committees for addressing questions related to controversies in clinical care. To ensure that research published complies with ethical research requirements, the journals seek statements about ethics approvals or consent, but verifying them by asking authors to provide copies of the same is not a common practice. Perhaps the journals trust that, given how the law works, institutions just won't permit unethical studies. However, this is not a safe assumption as lapses in enforcing ethical research standards may occur, particularly in elite entity environments where rapid innovation and reputational pressures can challenge existing oversight mechanisms, fostering an environment that may increase vulnerability to research integrity breaches.

The fundamental ethical principles are beneficence (promoting well-being), non-maleficence (not harming), autonomy (respecting participants' right to self-determination), and justice (fairness). The standard is to operationalize the implementation of these principles via an independent ethical review of a research proposal by a human research ethics committee, which should give formal approval before research begins. Obtaining individual participant consent is the standard for obtaining permission for the implementation of a research ethics committee approved project. Obtaining informed consent correctly isn't just a matter of simply asking for a signature on a form. Ethics committee approval and institutional research governance require that participants be fully informed using patient information sheets and other aids, such as a website with a greater written explanation or audio-visual material, which have been evaluated and approved by the committee. The consent must be entirely voluntary, and the information presented must be neutral and balanced. There should be no pressure. Journals can easily ask for authors to provide a copy of the signed and dated ethics committee approval letter and a copy of the unfilled or redacted consent form with patient information sheet as a safeguard. They can provide this information as a supplementary appendix with the published paper to reassure readers.

The established safeguards for participants in first-in-human procedures require strict compliance with ethical standards. The risk–benefit assessment should be informed by rigorous preclinical

Declaration of Helsinki: A living document on human research ethics produced and updated by the World Medical Association.

Principle: A value for guiding researchers' behavior.

Standard: Specification of the behavior that must be adhered to when carrying out research.

Human research ethics committee: Institutional Review Boards (IRB), set up under national research regulatory laws and tasked principally with the responsibility of giving formal approval to a research proposal and monitoring the ethical conduct of the research approved.

Power: The ability to influence others. The role asymmetry in a relationship permits the powerful to influence the vulnerable. The responsibility to prevent influence from turning into abuse lies with the powerful party.

evidence, independent ethical review, and fully informed voluntary consent to safeguard participants' human rights and prevent exploitation and harm. Yet, despite their global adoption and reinforcement through national regulations, enforcement at even the most prestigious institutions and journals can prove inadequate when innovation is prioritized over caution, creating conditions in which high-risk studies may advance without sufficient safeguards. The following case study illustrates this vulnerability through the trajectory of a 2011 publication that initially presented a novel approach but was later associated with concerns about compliance with ethical and research governance standards.

Shanghai ranking: Academic Ranking of World Universities, one of the most influential global research-based university rankings.

Impact factor: A journal statistic dividing the mean number of citations per article in a year by the total number of citable articles published in the previous two years.

A case study of alleged ethical failure, research misconduct, and patient harm

This case study summarizes information from publicly available investigation reports, court records, published retraction notices, and peer-reviewed publications, and discusses them in the context of research integrity scholarship.

Journal quartiles: A journal metric based on citation performance (e.g., impact factor, CiteScore, etc.) ranking all journals in a field into four equal groups, Q1–Q4.

In 2011, a research study detailing an innovative intervention was published in a leading medical journal. At the time of publication of this landmark article in 2011, the Karolinska Institute, Stockholm, Sweden, was one of the top institutions internationally, ranked 44th in the Shanghai Academic Ranking of World Universities. The Karolinska Institute is the same organization that is responsible for the committee for awarding the Nobel Prize in physiology or medicine to individuals who have made the most significant discoveries for the benefit of humankind in the biological and medical sciences. The article was published in *The Lancet* after peer review. The journal publisher was Elsevier, which is reported to be one of the world's largest publishers of scientific, technical, and medical literature with over 2500 academic journals. It had a journal impact factor of around 38, and it ranked second in Q1 among journals in the general and internal medicine category in 2011.

The paper's subtitle described the work as "a proof-of-concept study." It involved a single case report, a first-in-human study of the intervention, published following peer review (Box 10.1). The paper explicitly stated: "We obtained written informed consent from the patient, and the transplant procedure was approved by the local scientific ethics committee." There were around two dozen co-authors from Sweden, England, Iceland, and Germany, reflecting a collaborative international research effort with the lead and corresponding author affiliated with Karolinska. The authors' contributions section,

Peer review: Evaluation of scientific manuscripts by others working in the same field, invited by journal editors before acceptance for publication as definitive articles representing the version of record.

after describing individual inputs, stated that "all authors provided primary data for modelling scenarios, and assisted with interpretation of results and report revision." Earlier, the paper had been rejected following peer review by the *New England Journal of Medicine*. The paper's findings garnered attention for their implications in surgically treating a complex condition previously considered inoperable.

Box 10.1 Timeline of research integrity concerns: A case study of alleged ethical failure, research misconduct, and patient harm in Stockholm

Dates	Brief overview of events
2011	**Article submission, peer review, and publication** A paper was published in *The Lancet* following peer review. The paper stated that it "obtained written informed consent from the patient, and … was approved by the local scientific ethics committee." It had earlier been rejected by the *New England Journal of Medicine* with one peer reviewer commenting, "No papers are discussed from animal work performed by the author's group or other groups to support the success and long-term outcome of this experimental technique prior to translation into clinical practice? … Or was permission granted by the IRB …" *Source: DOI: 10.1016/S0140-6736(11)61715-7. URL: forbetterscience.com/2017/06/16/expert-review-macchiarini-papers-on-plastic-trachea-transplants-are-misconduct.*
2014	**Allegations of failure to obtain ethics committee approval and proper consent** A Retraction Watch blog reported that formal complaints covering several articles including the 2011 paper had been made alleging that the regional ethical review board approval had not been identified, and the consent had been obtained "17 days after," as well as there being data integrity concerns. *Source: URL: retractionwatch.com/2014/12/12/revealed-complaint-lodged-macchiarini-super-surgeon-investigation.*
2015	**Investigation** An editorial of *The Lancet* reported that the allegations of research misconduct were finally dismissed by an institutional investigation, after the *Nature* journal had initially reported that the misconduct had been found by an external investigator. *Sources: DOIs: 10.1038/nature.2015.17605; 10.1016/S0140-6736(15)00118-X.*

2016–18	**Expression of concern, institutional reopened investigation, and retraction** *The Experiments* (*Experimenten*), a three-part television documentary, aired in early 2016 repeated the research misconduct allegations. The institutional investigation was reopened. *The Lancet*'s 2016 expression of concern stated that there were "several new investigations into various aspects of the research." Several co-authors asked for their names to be removed from the 2011 paper. The Karolinska Institute misconduct investigation in 2018 found that ethical approvals were lacking, as was appropriate informed consent. Earlier external reviews in 2016 had also found weaknesses in the informed consent. The government dismissed the Karolinska Institute board. *The Lancet*'s 2018 retraction notice referred to "conclusions of the final investigation that has identified serious flaws in the conduct and reporting of this study. The report concludes there was scientific and ethical misconduct and requests retraction of the paper." Prosecution reopened criminal prosecution, having closed it a year earlier. *Sources: DOIs: 10.1016/S0140-6736(16)30114-3; 10.1016/S0140-6736(16)30091-5; 10.1016/S0140-6736(18)31558-7; 10.1038/nature.2016.19332; 10.1136/bmj.i4894. URLs: news.ki.se/media/109474/download; news.ki.se/news-archive/the-macchiarini-case-timeline; retractionwatch.com/2016/02/07/nobel-prize-official-resigns-in-wake-of-macchiarini-case; retractionwatch.com/2015/08/28/trachea-surgeon-macchiarini-acted-without-due-care-but-is-not-guilty-of-misconduct-karolinska; pubpeer.com/publications/89C5571232099E58F36E421E0DCEDD; news.ki.se/seven-researchers-responsible-for-scientific-misconduct-in-macchiarini-case.*
2020–23	**Institutional response and court judgment** In 2020, the institution introduced an action plan following the misconduct investigations. In 2023, the Swedish court reached an aggravated assault conviction (considering three cases including the patient in the 2011 paper) focused on disregarding known risks and lack of scientific basis (conditional intent). The *BMJ* journal reported that the court concluded that lead researcher was "aware but indifferent to the fact that the procedures would cause bodily harm and suffering." *Sources: DOI: 10.1136/bmj.p1442; URL: ki.se/en/about-ki/organisation-and-management/board-of-karolinska-institutet/action-plan-following-the-macchiarini-case-investigations.*

There were several papers involved; this chapter focuses on one paper, following it through in the timeline. See Box 10.2 for an outline of the research integrity roles of various actors in this case study and disclaimer.

Sources listed above are a few of the many that have covered this case study. This box summarizes reported allegations and findings; no judgment is intended.

By 2014, concerns began to emerge regarding the accuracy and completeness of the data presented in the study. Whistleblowers raised concerns about potential discrepancies in reporting patient outcomes, ethical approvals, consent, and the representation of results, as documented in formal complaints and subsequent investigations. These issues prompted an initial external investigation in 2015, which described shortcomings in research conduct, though a subsequent review at the institution led to clearance. However, ongoing scrutiny revealed inconsistencies, including questions about ethics committee approval and informed consent obtained after the procedures.

Retraction: Removing a published paper from the research record due, for example, to the discovery of a flaw in its integrity.

From 2016 to 2018, multiple probes deepened the examination of the research. A public television documentary and further complaints intensified the focus, resulting in the journal issuing an expression of concern in 2016 due to doubts about the work's integrity. The Karolinska Institute vice-chancellor resigned under pressure for having cleared the lead researcher of misconduct in 2015. Amid growing scrutiny and investigations into the paper's integrity, some co-authors requested name removals, including a whistleblower at Karolinska, as well as one co-author each from the University of Iceland and the University of Gothenburg, leading to a *Lancet* erratum in April 2016 that officially removed these three names from the author list. During the expression of concern process, additional co-authors sought to clarify or adjust their association with the paper, without formally requesting removal of their names.

Expression of concern: A note published by a journal to inform readers of there being the possibility of a concern about the integrity of a paper.

Erratum: A correction notice concerning a paper's version of record. It refers to the correction of a journal's error in the publishing process and is issued by the journal without the need for authors' approval. A **corrigendum** is a correction notice that requires approval by the authors.

The secretary general of the Nobel Prize assembly and committee for physiology or medicine resigned in 2016, as he expected to be a subject of the investigation into this case, and he wanted to avoid any effect on the award's reputation. Following the investigation, the Swedish government dismissed the entire Karolinska Institute board, citing findings that leadership had been described as negligent and indifferent. The government stated that a fresh start was needed to restore the institution's reputation. According to the definitive external investigation report, the institute was criticized for what was described as a "nonchalant attitude" toward laws and regulations, with concerns raised about leadership and a culture perceived as prioritizing excellence over ethical safeguards. It recognized that an "irresponsible attitude" to formalities at the institute increased "the risk of principal mistakes."

Box 10.2 Snapshot: The reported dimensions of research integrity issues in a case study of alleged ethical failure, research misconduct, and patient harm in Stockholm

Actors and their research integrity roles (described without assessing adequacy or compliance with standards)	**Reported observations over case study timeline** (no causal inference implied)
Institution: Karolinska Institute and its associated Karolinska University Hospital	
• Responsible for overseeing research conduct of their staff. • Responsible for differentiating between clinical practice and research by training staff who have dual roles and giving oversight to the work. • Responsible for investigating allegations of research misconduct under its policies and procedures. • Responsible for Nobel Prize assembly and committee in physiology or medicine.	• A 2011 article retracted after expression of concern and errata. • Resignation of the Nobel Prize secretary general. • Repeated multiple investigations. • Senior administration resignations. • The government dismissed the board of the Karolinska Institute. • Several other retractions and reports of research misconduct involving staff, as documented in public records. • Staff reportedly imprisoned following criminal proceedings related to the case. • University's Shanghai ranking decreased.
Journal: *The Lancet*, published by Elsevier	
• Responsible for editorial assessment and peer review of submitted manuscripts before publication. • Responsible for timely engagement in post-publication integrity concerns raised under journal editorial policies.	• A 2011 article retracted in 2018 after expression of concern and errata. • Additional retractions. • The journal impact factor increased, and quartile ranking was unchanged.
Funders: Various named in the 2011 paper	

• European Commission, Knut and Alice Wallenberg Foundation, Swedish Research Council, StratRegen, Vinnova Foundation, Radiumhemmet, Clinigene EU Network of Excellence, Swedish Cancer Society, Centre of Biosciences (The Live Cell imaging Unit), and UCL Business.	• No public comment noted.
Law courts	
• The courts examined the criminality of the research integrity failure.	• The lead researcher was given a prison sentence.
Whistleblowing and sleuthing	
• Sleuths made comments on PubPeer, For Better Science, and Retraction Watch after formal complaint has been filed by institutional whistleblowers who were co-authors of the paper.	• Mainstream media and medical journals covered the story. • Sleuths complained to the Swedish national research misconduct board.

See Box 1.1 for research integrity terminology.
See Box 1.2 for how research integrity concerns might arise and Box 1.3 for an outline of a research misconduct investigation.
See Box 10.1 for sources of information and the timeline of the case study.
Disclaimer: All factual statements are drawn from published literature and public records. No new allegation of research misconduct, dishonesty, or malice is intended or implied. The case study summarizes publicly available information and does not purport to determine liability or responsibility beyond what has been established in the cited records. References to individuals or organizations are made for academic discussion only and do not attribute intent or fault beyond the public record. When reporting changes in individual, institutional, organizational, and journal status or metrics, no causal inference is implied. The commentary and any opinions expressed are offered in good faith on matters of public interest concerning research integrity. Readers are encouraged to consult the original sources for full context.
University ranking data source: URL: www.shanghairanking.com/rankings/arwu/#### (year).
Journal impact factor and ranking are based on Journal Citation Reports.

PubPeer: An online platform for post-publication peer review.

The definitive investigation confirmed deviations from good research practices and that misconduct had occurred in several related papers, leading to a recommendation for retraction. According to the investigation report, responsibility was also assigned to some co-authors, including individuals who later raised concerns as whistleblowers. By 2018, *The Lancet* journal retracted the 2011 paper. Legal proceedings followed, with a court case in 2023 addressing charges related to the procedures' impact on three patients, including the case reported in the 2011 *Lancet* paper. All three patients had died. The appeals court ruled that the actions constituted aggravated assault, emphasizing the foreseeable risks and indifference to potential harm, resulting in a prison sentence of two and a half years, marking a significant judicial outcome in a case involving medical innovation, research ethics, and accountability.

Court records show that the lead researcher received a prison sentence in 2023 and, as of early 2026, was serving the term following exhaustion of appeals. Publicly available bibliometric indicators of the lead researcher's *h*-index could not be verified in 2025; the reasons for this were not publicly documented. The 2011 paper had been cited around 500 times in total before retraction, according to Google Scholar. The Karolinska Institute maintained its top ranking standing at 50th position in the Shanghai Academic Ranking of World Universities in 2025 (Box 10.2). The recent *Lancet* journal impact factor was around 88, and it ranked first (Q1) among journals in the category of general and internal medicine, whereas it had ranked second in 2011. Changes in institutional rankings, article-level citations, academic indices, or journal metrics are reported descriptively only; no causal relationship with the case study is asserted or implied.

h(Hirsh)-index: A popular statistic to measure scientific output, taking account of citations, e.g., an *h*-index of 5 means that the author has 5 published papers that have been cited 5 times or more.

Google Scholar: A freely accessible web search engine that indexes scholarly literature across a wide range of formats and disciplines, aggregating nearly all major scholarly publishing.

Root cause analysis: Institutional culture

Drawing from the investigation reports, court judgment, and public records summarized above, the following analysis examines the institutional and systemic factors that contribute to the research integrity culture. Analyses of this case study in scholarly commentary have emphasized the role of institutional culture and oversight structures in shaping research practices. Rather than a single root cause, a constellation of factors may have influenced how integrity concerns were identified and addressed.

CRediT: Contributor Roles Taxonomy is a system for classifying the roles played by individual authors and those acknowledged in a scholarly publication.

The case study has been cited as revealing significant weaknesses in institutional oversight mechanisms, particularly in research oversight, consent, and patient protections. Other case studies of ethical failures are covered in Chapters 4 and 12. In this case study, questions were raised about how high-risk intervention research proceeded without a documented independent research ethics board's risk–benefit assessment. Similarly, informed consent processes appeared to be flawed, with the forms signed retrospectively after surgery had been completed. Investigators considered these lapses inconsistent with fundamental ethical standards, such as those outlined in the Declaration of Helsinki, which demand robust preclinical data and clear participant autonomy before first-in-human studies. The absence of such safeguards not only raised serious patient safety concerns but also un-

Accountability: A responsible research principle guiding individuals and organizations to be answerable for the research they engage in from idea to post-publication.

dermined the integrity of the research environment, contributing to concerns that innovation may have been prioritized over regulatory compliance. The institution had existing integrity and ethical policies; however, investigations raised concerns that these policies were insufficiently enforced or inadequate in scope, lacking robust checks for high-risk research, unclear leadership accountability, non-systematic research ethics training, and unintegrated support systems. Commentators suggested that institutional emphasis on scientific prestige may have influenced decision-making, raising concerns about whether patient safety safeguards were sufficiently prioritized. The government sacked the entire board and a new action plan for a fresh start emphasized training, incident reporting, and accountability for moving towards an integrity culture (Box 10.3). The government in 2020 also shifted investigations of serious research misconduct from individual universities to an independent national agency. The goal was to ensure transparent, impartial handling and restore public trust in research after the scandal exposed flaws in self-regulation. Two further papers related to this case study were retracted by *The Lancet* in 2023 following a whistleblower-triggered investigation by the Swedish national research misconduct board (DOI: 10.1016/S0140-6736(08)61598-6; 10.1016/S0140-6736(13)62033-4).

Box 10.3 Some recommendations for institutions arising from the Karolinska action plan

Feature	Comments
Research integrity orientation	• Comprehensive research integrity webpages with guidelines. • Mandatory research integrity trainings for students and staff, especially supervisors. • Mandatory laboratory safety training. • Research integrity as an integral part of induction of new employees. • Strong research training leadership for the educational program covering ethics, standards, laws, and regulations.
Support for senior leadership	• Training for senior administrators and executives on legal responsibilities and work environment. • Work environment coordination agreements between hospital and university.

Research governance		• Council for audit of compliance with good research practice to feedback directly to senior administrative leadership. • Anonymous whistleblowing policies. • Quality assurance with audits and inspections. • Mandatory research integrity breach incident reporting and documentation. • National authority for assessments of allegations of serious research misconduct.

Sources: DOI: 10.1016/j.respol.2018.03.020. URL: ki.se/en/about-ki/organisation-and-management/board-of-karolinska-institutet/action-plan-following-the-macchiarini-case-investigations.

Authorship accountability emerged as another critical shortfall, with the original publication listing numerous collaborators from multiple European institutions. As scrutiny intensified, several co-authors on the 2011 paper sought to remove their names, highlighting challenges related to collective responsibility in large collaborative authorship. This pattern reflects broader challenges in large-scale collaborative research, where diffuse accountability can dilute ethical vigilance. The topic of collective authorship accountability has been debated in the literature (DOI: 10.1089/scd.2018.0214) (Chapter 9). From a research integrity perspective, the journal publishing the 2011 article may be considered to have missed an opportunity to verify essential documentation, such as human research ethics committee approval and consent forms, prior to publication. Prestigious outlets, in their gatekeeping role, are expected to demand evidence of compliance, but in this instance, initial rapid acceptance and delayed retractions may have contributed to the continued circulation of findings later questioned in investigations, potentially amplifying harm to the scientific record and public trust.

Internationally, in many research environments, there can be strong incentives to pursue prestigious and groundbreaking findings. The reflection and institutional response of Karolinska have been widely discussed as an instructive example for the broader research community. A comprehensive research integrity action plan focusing on strengthened ethical and professional training, leadership support, enhanced documentation systems, whistleblower policies, misconduct prevention, and independent impartial investigations should be in place at all institutions. Ultimately, these reforms represent a commitment to cultural transformation, emphasizing transparency and accountability to prevent recurrence. Rebuilding trust requires sustained vigilance. The case study has been widely cited as a cautionary example that underscores the importance of consistent enforcement of research integrity standards. As presented here, it illustrates how complex interactions between innovation, governance, and accountability can give rise to significant research integrity concerns documented in investigations and commentaries. The chapter underscores the importance of sustained attention to ethical standards in research integrity.

Chapter 10: Institutional research culture: Alleged ethical failure and patient harm in Stockholm – Key points

Advice for researchers

- Prioritize rigorous preclinical evidence before any first-in-human application, ensuring that interventions rest on a solid scientific foundation. There should be no rush to perform unproven, high-risk experiments without adequate safeguards.
- Uphold personal accountability in collaborative authorship; detailed contribution statements and ongoing responsibility for published work help prevent later disassociation when issues arise (also see Chapter 9).
- Foster a culture of open internal critique and early reporting of concerns, recognizing that ethical vigilance strengthens rather than undermines scientific progress. Do this despite the risk that whistleblowing may expose you to being implicated in the misconduct reported.
- Do not bypass ethics and consent standards. Document human research ethics committee approval, making signed and dated letters publicly available (see also Chapters 4 and 12 concerning alleged ethical failures).
- Document informed consent meticulously and prospectively, transparently communicating all known risks to maintain participant autonomy and trust.

Recommendations for journals and publishers

- Strengthen pre-publication verification of essential ethics documentation, including signed and dated human research ethics committee approval letters and evidence of proper consent processes with consent form and patient information sheet. Move this process from verification to public disclosure by including these documents as supplementary material with the published papers (also see Chapters 4 and 12 concerning documentation of human research ethics committee approval as an integrity check).

- Train editors and peer reviewers in making assessments of compliance with ethical approval and consent standards.
- Implement mandatory use of standardized authorship contribution frameworks, e.g., CRediT (DOI: 10.21037/atm.2019.12.96), to clarify responsibilities and to help reduce diffuse accountability.
- Publish peer review comments and authors' responses with papers, moving to open peer review with open identities.
- Respond swiftly and transparently to post-publication concerns, using expressions of concern and retractions as necessary to protect the scientific record.
- Balance the drive for publication of impactful innovation with robust gatekeeping, ensuring that editorial processes prioritize participant protection and research integrity over headline potential.

Open peer review: An umbrella term for the various options available to make peer review compatible with open science principles.

Roles of institutions and funders

- Organizational culture is the foundation on which research compliant with international standards, such as the Declaration of Helsinki, is conducted. Embed comprehensive research integrity training for researchers as well as senior administration (Box 10.3).
- Prioritize patient safety, particularly for high-risk translational work. Ensure that first-in-human studies are carried out with a proper preclinical foundation.
- Adequately resource human research ethics committees to undertake their functions.
- Establish anonymous incident reporting to support whistleblowers (Box 1.2).
- Establish clear, independent mechanisms for handling misconduct allegations, avoiding conflicts of interest, and ensuring impartial follow-through (Box 1.3).
- Funders should require explicit milestones for preclinical validation and ethical compliance in translational grants, tying continued support to adherence to clear go/no-go criteria for progression to first-in-human studies.

Research culture: The academic environment comprising the norms, values, expectations, attitudes, and behaviors within research organizations. Academic freedom, collegiality, collaboration, equality and diversity, research integrity (ethics and professionalism), conflict management with openness, accountability, and transparency are all features of the research culture.

11 *Copy-paste without citation*

Allegations of plagiarism in a British journal

Research integrity: Undertaking research and publication following ethical and professional principles and standards. Responsible research and publication practices pave the way for science to be regarded as trustworthy. Integrity failures may result from honest errors or deliberate misconduct.

Plagiarism, the copying of another's work without attribution, is one of the most serious breaches of academic integrity, undermining trust in the scientific record. A former editor-in-chief of the *British Journal of Sports Medicine* (2001–2008) wrote several single-authored editorials, opinion pieces, commentaries, and letters, which became the subject of allegations concerning editorial practices in BMJ medical publishing. To begin with, a 2005 editorial, later found to have plagiarized a 2000 Physics World article, was retracted in 2022. Independent scrutiny by research integrity commentators identified multiple instances of a writing pattern that was characterized in subsequent reports as plagiarism, self-plagiarism, and misrepresentation. Comprehensive publisher investigations were undertaken in response to formal complaints by an author whose work was copied without attribution, and the input of sleuths and the institution to which the editor was affiliated. Publisher investigations resulted in over a dozen additional single-author publications being retracted, as documented in official notices. Furthermore, the publisher placed expressions of concern on 74 articles, according to its public record. This case study illustrates systemic vulnerabilities in editorial oversight, the critical role of whistleblowing and sleuthing, and the shared responsibility of journals and institutions in safeguarding research integrity. This chapter will highlight the reputational consequences of misconduct for individuals and organizations, offering a cautionary example for medical publishing.

A victim of plagiarism

Plagiarism (Latin root plagium means kidnapping) is the copying of the work of other authors, including text, tables, images, data, or other intellectual property, and presenting it as if it were one's own work without proper citation to the original source or without formally obtaining permission. Self-plagiarism is the recycling of one's own previously published text without attribution, giving the impression of new content when it is not. Text recycling is sometimes a term used to describe self-plagiarism. Duplication is also a form of self-plagiarism, describing the republication of an entire article without identifying

DOI: 10.1201/9781003655916-11

the original. Note that republication with the source article identified is often used in the context of the need for dissemination and translations; this practice is not plagiarism. Misrepresentation, a form distinct from plagiarism, is the incorrect or misleading use of another author's words or ideas in a way that distorts their original meaning. Since the mid-2000s, journals have been deploying automated plagiarism checks, and with this intervention, the copy-pasting of text without attribution has been controlled in submissions. Automated checks have also allowed post-publication scrutiny, leading to allegations, investigations, retractions, and corrections for various forms of plagiarism (Box 11.1).

Plagiarism: Copying the work of others (text, tables, images, data, etc.) and presenting it as one's own work without proper citation to the source.

Box 11.1 Harvard university plagiarism review and resignation of its president

Background

- A new Harvard University president, with an illustrious record including education at Princeton, Stanford, and Harvard, took office in mid 2023.
- In late 2023, allegations of plagiarism emerged concerning plagiarism in her academic work, focusing on her 1997 PhD dissertation and several published articles. One published allegation concerning the thesis stated that it "lifts an entire paragraph nearly verbatim … does provide a reference to the original authors, she uses their verbatim language, with a few trivial synonym substitutions, without providing quotation marks."

Investigation

- The university conducted an internal investigation, demonstrating accountability amid academic and political scrutiny.
- An eight-page report to the United States House Committee on Education was made public.
- The report acknowledged instances of textual overlap and inadequate citation, but concluded these did not rise to the level of formal research misconduct under Harvard's policies.
- The university noted that the president had already submitted corrections to some works to address citation issues.

Outcome

- The president resigned within a year of appointment, following public controversy and scrutiny over plagiarism allegations.

Sources: DOIs: 10.1007/s10928-024-09904-z. URLs: www.city-journal.org/article/is-claudine-gay-a-plagiarist; www.thecrimson.com/article/2023/12/12/allegations-plagiarism-gay-dissertation; www.harvard.edu/media-relations/wp-content/uploads/sites/3/2024/01/Harvards-Detailed-Description-of-its-Review-Process.pdf; www.independent.co.uk/news/ap-mit-boston-elise-stefanik-republican-b2482877.html.

In the context of academic or scholarly publishing, an author whose work has been plagiarized can be described as a victim of plagiarism. Victim is an accurate description of the injured party because the loss of recognition of the original author due to the lack of proper attribution is a form of harm suffered. It is not just in the form of abuse or misappropriation of intellectual property, but in terms of lost citations, also a loss in terms of diminished scholarly impact, which in turn has professional and reputational consequences. Many plagiarized authors also describe feeling insulted, disrespected, or exploited when their work is copied without credit. Protecting oneself from becoming prey to plagiarism is an impossible task. Scientists rely entirely on the scientific and publishing community's integrity in this regard.

Journal: An establishment composed of editors and other publishing staff who organize the peer review of manuscripts and their publication.

Plagiarism, when found to be intentional, is widely regarded as one of the most serious breaches of academic integrity. It raises questions about the effectiveness of existing detection and prevention mechanisms within journals and institutions. At its core, as it involves misappropriation of intellectual ownership, it undermines trust in the scientific record and diminishes the rightful recognition of original authors. Beyond plagiarism in its various forms, misrepresentation of sources also distorts the literature, misleading readers about the originality or evidentiary basis of claims. The responsibility to safeguard against these practices lies not only with individual authors but also with journals and publishers. Journals are expected to implement robust screening mechanisms, including plagiarism detection software. Publishers must ensure that allegations are investigated promptly. Editors, in particular, carry a dual responsibility: they must uphold the highest standards in their own publications while also serving as gatekeepers for the work of others. When editors themselves engage in plagiarism, the breach is especially damaging, as it compromises both the integrity of the journal and the broader trust in scientific publishing.

Institution: An academic organization, typically a university, where research takes place. It has the responsibility to oversee ethical and professional research conduct.

Publisher: An organization whose business is to prepare and issue works, such as books, magazines, journals, etc., for public distribution. It has the responsibility to oversee ethical and professional publication conduct.

A case study of concern about editorial practices

This case study summarizes information from publicly available blogs, published retraction notices, peer-reviewed publications, and PubPeer comments, and discusses them in the context of research integrity scholarship.

In 2005, a single-authored editorial was published in a British sports medicine journal that was considered a rising star in its academic category. The author was the journal's chief editor at the time of

Shanghai Ranking: Academic Ranking of World Universities, one of the most influential global research-based university rankings.

publication. His institution was the University of Melbourne, which ranked 82nd in the Shanghai Academic Ranking of World Universities. The journal was the BMJ publishers' *British Journal of Sports Medicine* or *BJSM*. BMJ is a leading publisher of medical journals, owned by the British Medical Association. Headquartered in London, it publishes, including the BMJ, more than 60 journals. *BJSM* had a journal impact factor of around 2, and it ranked in the Q3 quartile among journals in the sports medicine category in 2005 (Box 11.2). The single-author 2005 editorial later became the focus of plagiarism allegations.

An article had appeared in 2000 in *Physics World*, a monthly magazine published by the Institute of Physics, a professional society for physicists, headquartered in London, United Kingdom. Substantial portions of this magazine article had been copied and pasted without attribution in the 2005 *BJSM* editorial (Box 11.3). The author of the *Physics World* article recognized the plagiarism of his work for the first time in 2012–2013 and informed the magazine, but nothing happened then, according to his own website. In the years that followed, he learned about what ought to be done about plagiarism in academic publishing when working as a conference proceedings editor. In 2021, he complained to the *BJSM*, which forwarded the concern raised to the BMJ publication integrity office for investigation. The 2005 *BJSM* article was retracted in 2022. According to public reports, the author also resigned from his role as an expert in a professional body. This was the first formal trigger for scrutiny of the author's publication record. After the complaint about the 2005 article became known, a sleuth began systematically examining other single-authored publications of the former *BJSM* editor and identified multiple cases of plagiarism. There were repeated instances of text recycling and unattributed copying across single-authored *BJSM* editorials. The BMJ investigations reported multiple findings that were characterized as plagiarism, duplication, and misrepresentation in official notices. According to these findings, the conduct met the BMJ journals' definition of plagiarism. *BJSM* announced nine further retractions: five for plagiarism, three for duplicate publication, and one for misrepresentation. At the same time, BMJ placed expressions of concern on all his 74 single-author papers.

The case did not end there. In 2023–2024, the University of Melbourne, to which the editor was affiliated, requested *BJSM* to review additional articles. This led to further retractions. The university's actions, as reported, illustrate how institutions may engage with journals when concerns are raised. The case overall illustrates how external whistleblowing, journal investigations, and institutional pressure combined to bring to light the issues documented in retrac-

Impact factor: A journal statistic dividing the mean number of citations per article in a year by the total number of citable articles published in the previous two years.

Retraction: Removing a published paper from the research record due, for example, to the discovery of a flaw in its integrity.

Expression of concern: A note published by a journal to inform readers of there being the possibility of a concern about the integrity of a paper.

Sleuthing: Investigation of possible research and publication misconduct and questionable practices by volunteer researchers.

h(Hirsh)-index: A popular statistic to measure scientific output, taking account of citations, e.g., an *h*-index of 5 means that the author has 5 published papers that have been cited 5 times or more.

tion notices. Publicly available bibliometric indicator of the former editor's *h*-index was around 100 in 2025, according to Research.com. The University of Melbourne ranked at 38th position in the Shanghai Academic Ranking of World Universities in 2025, having risen from 82nd in 2005. The recent *BJSM* journal impact factor was around 11, and it ranked in the Q1 quartile among journals in the category of sports medicine, whereas it had ranked in the Q3 quartile in 2005. Changes in institutional rankings, academic indices, or journal metrics are reported descriptively only; no causal relationship with the case study is asserted or implied.

Journal quartiles: A journal metric based on citation performance (e.g., impact factor, CiteScore, etc.) ranking all journals in a field into four equal groups, Q1–Q4.

Box 11.2 Timeline of research integrity concerns: A case study of alleged plagiarism in a British journal

Dates	Brief overview of events
2000	**Original article publication** A magazine article appeared in *Physics World*, published by the United Kingdom Institute of Physics. *Source: URL: physicsworld.com/a/physics-technology-and-the-olympics.*
2005	**Single-authored editorial published in the *British Journal of Sports Medicine*** The author was the chief editor of *BJSM*. *Source: DOI: 10.1136/bjsports/39/11/785.long.ret.*
2012–13	**Initial concern** The original author, having come across plagiarizing of his work, informed the original publisher, but nothing happened, according to the author's public account. *Source: URL: stevehaake.com/news/paul-mccrory-plagiarism-row.*
2021–22	**Formal complaint to *BJSM*, investigation, and retraction of the editorial** A complaint made to the journal was passed on to the publisher BMJ for investigation. According to the affected author, "over half of the words in the article were mine (50.7% to be exact): that's 560 words copied and pasted." The retraction notice stated: "This article has been retracted due to unlawful and indefensible breach of copyright. There was significant overlap with a previous publication …" According to public reports, the author resigned from his role as an expert in a professional sports organization. *Sources: URL: retractionwatch.com/2022/02/28/this-is-frankly-insulting-an-author-plagiarized-by-a-journal-editor-speaks; www.the-scientist.com/neurologist-paul-mccrory-resigns-amid-plagiarism-allegations-69778.*

2022	**Further allegations, comprehensive investigation, and further retractions** On the completion of the overarching investigation, there were nine single-author opinion pieces, commentaries, and editorials retracted including "five cases of plagiarism and three of redundant publication … the other retracted article … inaccurately quotes and misrepresents ..." There were expressions of concern placed on 74 of the editor's single-authored papers. There was an independent review conducted by the professional sports organization where the author served as an expert. *Sources: DOI:* 10.1136/bmj.o2442. *URL: resources.afl.com.au/afl/document/2022/10/25/8fdd50b6-98a4-47db-9f71-3d5d0e42fa9c/Final_Report_171022.pdf.*
2023–24	**Institutional request for further investigation by BMJ** At the institution's request, according to BMJ statements, the journal retracted further papers. The total number of retractions reached 17, including three for duplicate publication or self-plagiarism, and two other articles were corrected for "inappropriate reuse of content," which is another form of self-plagiarism. *Sources: DOI:* 10.1136/bjsports-2022-106408; *URLs: bjsm.bmj.com/content/56/23/1327.responses; bmjgroup.com/journal-retracts-6-further-articles-and-corrects-2-others-authored-by-former-editor; www.eurekalert.org/news-releases/1043822.*

There were several papers involved; this chapter focuses on one paper, following it through in the timeline. See Box 11.3 for an outline of the research integrity roles of various actors in this case study and disclaimer. Sources listed above are a few of the many that have covered this case study. This box summarizes reported allegations and findings; no judgment is intended.

Box 11.3 Snapshot: The dimensions of research integrity issues in a case study of alleged plagiarism in a British journal

Actors and their research integrity roles (described without assessing adequacy or compliance with standards)	**Reported observations over case study timeline** (no causal inference implied)
Institution: University of Melbourne	
• Responsible for overseeing research conduct of its staff. • Responsible for investigating allegations of research misconduct under its policies and procedures. • Had affiliated with it an institute where the lead author of the retracted article was based. • Requested publisher investigation.	• A 2005 article retracted • Multiple expressions of concern. • Institute distanced itself from the retractions. • Publisher investigations. • Lead researcher resignation from expert role in a professional organization. • University'sShanghairankingincreased.

Journal: *British Journal of Sports Medicine*, published by BMJ Group of the British Medical Association	
• Publisher responsible for the publishing infrastructure of its journals • Has ultimate responsibility for enforcing policies on publishing integrity • Responsible for oversight of editors' work. • Responsible for plagiarism checks.	• A 2005 article retracted. • Multiple expressions of concern. • Additional retractions. • The journal impact factor and quartile ranking increased.
Sleuthing	
• Sleuths made investigations after a formal complaint had been had led to retraction of a 2005 paper.	• Mainstream media and top medical journals covered the story.

See Box 1.1 for research integrity terminology.
See Box 1.2 for how research integrity concerns might arise and Box 1.3 for an outline of a research misconduct investigation.
See Box 11.2 for sources of information and the timeline of the case study.
Disclaimer: All factual statements are drawn from published literature and public records. No new allegation of research misconduct, dishonesty, or malice is intended or implied. The case study summarizes publicly available information and does not purport to determine liability or responsibility beyond what has been established in the cited records. References to individuals or organizations are made for academic discussion only and do not attribute intent or fault beyond the public record. When reporting changes in individual, institutional, organizational, and journal status or metrics, no causal inference is implied. The commentary and any opinions expressed are offered in good faith on matters of public interest concerning research integrity. Readers are encouraged to consult the original sources for full context.
University ranking data source: URL: www.shanghairanking.com/rankings/arwu/#### (year).
Journal impact factor and ranking are based on Journal Citation Reports.

Respect for intellectual ownership

Drawing from the case study above, the following discussion examines the responsibilities of readers, journals, and institutions in responding to suspected plagiarism, and offers guidance for safeguarding integrity in scientific writing.

COPE: Committee on Publication Ethics issues guidance to journals on responsible publication practices, including handling research misconduct allegations.

Readership plays a role in safeguarding the integrity of scientific writing. If someone suspects that their own work, or that of another author, has been plagiarized, they ought to be prepared to act. The appropriate course is to document the overlap clearly and report it to the appropriate organization, i.e., the journal containing the plagiarized text in its article or its publisher's integrity office, or in case of plagiarism in a master's or doctoral thesis, the research integrity office of the degree-awarding institution. Raising concerns should be done professionally, with side-by-side comparisons of the texts in question. The Committee on Publication Ethics (COPE) advises publishers to treat plagiarism as a serious integrity breach, investigate all allegations systematically, and respond proportionately depending on the severity. Journals are therefore obliged to investigate such complaints formally, and complainants should expect transparent communication about the outcome. Delay in handling concerns or informality may allow integrity issues to remain unresolved.

Plagiarism, whether intentional or inadvertent, remains one of the most corrosive threats to the credibility of academic writing. The case study explored in this chapter demonstrates how concerns related to research writing integrity may remain unaddressed for extended periods before being identified. The case prompted wide discussion across research communities, journals, publishers, and institutions. It reminds us that vigilance is not optional but essential, and that integrity must be actively safeguarded at every stage of the academic writing and publication process. For authors, the challenge is twofold: to avoid deliberate appropriation of other authors' works and to guard against unintentional lapses in citation, paraphrasing, or text recycling.

Generative Artificial Intelligence: AI can be deployed to draft and revise manuscripts, among other possibilities. Its use should be transparently reported without being credited in authorship.

While the case study above concerns traditional plagiarism, the rise of generative AI (Artificial Intelligence) introduces new dimensions to the challenge of maintaining originality and attribution in scientific writing. Generative Pretrained Transformer, or ChatGPT, is one such AI tool. While AI can assist with paraphrasing, grammar, and similarity checks, its outputs must be verified, disclosed, and used responsibly (Box 11.4). Far from replacing human accountability, AI underscores the need for authors to remain vigilant stewards of originality and accuracy. Transparency, accountability, and respect for intellectual ownership in academic writing should be an integral part of research integrity training. Reflection on documented plagiarism case studies should be a part of such training to strengthen safeguards through the study of real-world examples. Disclosure of AI use, as emphasized in recent research guidances, is not a confession but a routine part of transparent scholarly reporting.

ChatGPT: A generative AI tool that may be deployed to draft and revise manuscripts, among other scientific tasks. Its role should be explicitly disclosed.

Accountability: A responsible research principle guiding individuals and organizations to be answerable for the research they engage in from idea to post-publication.

This chapter underscores that integrity in publishing is a collective responsibility. Publishers, journals, and editors must uphold clear standards, apply plagiarism detection tools judiciously, and respond transparently when concerns arise. Institutions, in turn, carry the responsibility of embedding integrity into research writing training, ensuring that plagiarism is avoided and misconduct is addressed. Together, these actors form the ecosystem of accountability that sustains trust in science. By learning from past cases and adapting to new challenges such as AI, the academic community can strengthen its safeguards and reaffirm its commitment to honesty, transparency, and respect for intellectual ownership. Building on these reflections, the following key points distill practical lessons for researchers, journals, publishers, and institutions, offering clear guidance on how integrity can be safeguarded in everyday scholarly practice.

Box 11.4 Some recommendations for responsible use of generative AI (Artificial Intelligence) in scientific writing

Feature	Comments
Accountability	Authors remain responsible for the text drafted when AI is used. AI-generated text should not be considered anything more than unverified notes for manuscript writing. AI cannot be an author as cannot take responsibility for the work.
Verification	Undertake fact-checking, source validation, and plagiarism screening of AI-assisted drafts.
Attribution	AI does not inherently follow citation formating norms; authors must insert and check references.
Bias	There is a possiblity of hidden bias in AI-generated drafts depending on availability of sources; authors remain responsible for capturing the relevant sources.
Paraphrasing	Text recycling can happen in paraphrased passages; for reducing the risk of unintentional plagiarism, always compare with the original to check accuracy of text and citation to ensure that the meaning is preserved and sources are cited correcty.
Quotation accuracy	When using AI to detect where direct quotations might be appropriate, verify wording against the original source for exact phrasing.
Misrepresentation	AI may paraphrase or quote in way that changes the original meaning; authors remain responsbile for avoiding misrepresentation.
Similarity checks	Run AI-assisted drafts through plagiarism detection tools to identify inadvertent overlaps.

Disclosure	Authors must verify all AI-assisted content, including checking facts, drafting text, generating figures, summarizing literature, genrating references, avoiding retracted citations, etc. Disclose transparently the AI tool, version, how it was used, and affirm that the human authors take responsibility for the final content.

Sources: DOI: 10.1080/0142159X.2025.2607513. URLs: publicationethics.org/guidance/cope-position/authorship-and-ai-tools; www.sagepub.com/about/sage-policies/corporate-policies/ai-author-guidelines.
Note: This guidance does not pertain to performing peer review and editorial assessment of submitted manuscripts, for which reviewers and editors should receive guidance from publisher.

Chapter 11: Copy-paste without citation: Allegations of plagiarism in a British journal – Key points

Advice for researchers

- Ensure that scientific writing cites properly, free from plagiarism or text recycling.
- Respect sources, quoting, and referencing accurately; misrepresentation of prior work undermines credibility.
- Disclose overlaps with previous publications and avoid duplicate submissions (Box 9.1). As well as avoiding plagiarism, this is important for transparency in authorship.
- Use generative AI responsibly with transparent disclosures (Box 11.4).

Recommendations for journals and publishers

- Define plagiarism clearly in instructions to authors and in the journal policies.
- Implement robust similarity checks, using plagiarism detection software, in all submissions. Communicate neutrally when contacting authors about the findings of similarity checks, explaining the journal's position and requesting clarification.
- Ensure that the similarity check reports are evaluated reasonably, recognizing that text matches can legitimately come from methods outlined in published protocols, references, etc. Assess the reported similarity percentages by cross-checking against sources of overlap. There is no single uni-

versally acceptable numerical percentage threshold interpretable without qualitative assessment.
- Be judicious in differentiating severity, e.g., clear plagiarism when there are large unattributed portions of text or data (requiring rejection or retraction); redundancy or self-plagiarism with reuse of small amounts of the author's own work (may be resolved with revision or correction); or minor overlap or short phrases, especially from non-native speakers (may be acceptable).
- Editors are expected to uphold the same standards they enforce on others; departures from these standards at the editorial level are widely regarded as particularly damaging to trust in publishing. Publishers should undertake audits for editorial accountability.
- Provide clear editorial policies and training on plagiarism handling. Publishers should apply the same standards across all journals to maintain credibility.
- Respond promptly to complaints via publisher-led investigations, publish clear retraction notices, and correct errors in reporting. Investigate comprehensively, as older publications with plagiarism may surface years later (Box 1.3).

Roles of institutions and funders

- Instill integrity in the scientific writing culture, promote intellectual honesty, and provide clear policies, procedures, and support.
- Provide support, e.g., plagiarism detection software, and training, e.g., paraphrasing, attribution, and case studies of plagiarism, to all researchers preparing submissions and theses.
- Ensure training in research integrity makes it clear that plagiarism is unacceptable in any form, taking into account the implications of the use of artificial intelligence in science writing
- Establish whistleblowing policies, so staff feel empowered to report suspected plagiarism (Box 1.2).
- Universities and research institutions should review allegations thoroughly and request publisher-led investigations when needed (Box 1.3).
- Funders should check for plagiarism in grant applications submitted.

12 *Professional regulatory investigation*

Alleged ethical concerns and conflict non-disclosure in London

Professional regulatory bodies, statutory organizations that ensure health practitioners meet standards of competence and conduct, exist to protect the public. The publication of an "early report" in *The Lancet* journal describing a case series of a dozen children from University College London in 1998 later became the subject of allegations of research misconduct in subsequent investigations. Within the evidence-based medicine hierarchy, this type of study represented the lowest form of evidence; however, it suggested a possible relationship between exposure to the measles, mumps, and rubella (MMR) vaccination and autism. Extensive media coverage of this claim was followed by a public health impact, with vaccine hesitancy associated with UK MMR uptake dropping from over 90% at the time of publication to approximately 80% by 2003–2004, contributing to measles outbreaks. Allegations of research misconduct first came to light via independent investigative journalism in 2004, reporting previously undisclosed financial conflicts of interest, highlighting the critical role of external investigative reporting versus internal academic vigilance. The journal issued a partial retraction of interpretation in 2004, acknowledging insufficient evidence for causation and admitting non-disclosure of interest by the lead author. *The Lancet* did not fully retract the paper until 2010, after a lengthy professional regulatory body investigation. The institution and journal were criticized in public commentary and subsequent reviews for their handling of initial concerns. Investigations and regulatory findings in this case raised concerns regarding research ethics committee approval, consent procedures, disclosure of financial interests, participant recruitment, and the accuracy of reported clinical information. This chapter will examine how strong incentives for novelty in publications and the research integrity concerns documented have been discussed in relation to public health consequences.

Research integrity: Undertaking research and publication following ethical and professional principles and standards. Responsible research and publication practices pave the way for science to be regarded as trustworthy. Integrity failures may result from honest errors or deliberate misconduct.

Institution: An academic organization, typically a university, where research takes place. It has the responsibility to oversee ethical and professional research conduct.

Professional regulatory body: By law, healthcare professionals must be registered with a professional regulatory body to ensure they are fit and licensed to practice.

DOI: 10.1201/9781003655916-12

Professional regulation and research integrity

Professional regulatory bodies related to healthcare exist to ensure that the public is protected from the risks associated with the work of health professionals, including doctors, nurses, pharmacists, physiotherapists, radiographers, etc. For this, they must ensure that health professionals are fit and licensed to practice. Health professional regulation also covers, in alphabetical order, biomedical scientists, chiropractors, clinical scientists, dentists, dental nurses and technicians, dietitians, hearing aid dispensers, midwives, nursing associates, occupational therapists, operating department practitioners, opticians, osteopaths, paramedics, and speech and language therapists, among others.

Regulator of medicines: A formal body set up for official approvals of drugs and devices, e.g., Food and Drug Administration (FDA), European Medicines Agency (EMA), etc.

The term professional regulatory body should not be confused with the term regulator of medicines used in this book for a formal body set up for official approvals of drugs and devices, e.g., European Medicines Agency (EMA). The professional regulatory body's role is to ensure that registered professionals meet the standards of competence and conduct. This is achieved through a statutory framework that maintains a register of qualified practitioners. The regulatory body sets a code of ethical and professional practice. Against this code deployed as a standard, the regulatory body investigates fitness to practice concerns raised, which may include allegations of research misconduct. The body imposes sanctions when standards are breached. Unlike voluntary non-profit societies or associations, regulators have legal enforcement powers, focusing on patient safety, public trust, and accountability rather than advocacy or representation.

Ethics: Decision-making based on moral values that distinguish between right and wrong.

Principle: A value for guiding researchers' behavior.

Standard: Specification of the behavior that must be adhered to when carrying out research.

The code of practice documented by the professional regulatory bodies includes an emphasis on evidence-based practice to reduce harm from unproven practices and engagement in research to reduce uncertainty in evidence. Adhering to principles like human research ethics committee review, informed consent, and transparency, e.g., declaring conflicts of interest, is all part of the honesty and integrity required by professional codes. Professional regulatory bodies, in addition to institutions and journals, may also investigate allegations of research misconduct. The professional body's role becomes important when, for instance, including patients in research without human research ethics committee approval or data falsification or fabrication may impair a health professional's fitness to practice or compromise public trust in the profession. This reinforces that research is integral to quality healthcare service delivery. Extreme cases of research misconduct can lead to erasure from the professional register.

Human research ethics committee: Institutional Review Boards (IRB), set up under national research regulatory laws and tasked principally with the responsibility of giving formal approval to a research proposal and monitoring the ethical conduct of the research approved.

This chapter covers a case study where a professional regulatory body undertook a fitness to practice investigation upon being alerted about a research integrity concern and identified failures in ethical safeguards and conflict disclosure, information ultimately used by the publishing journal for retracting a paper.

A case study of alleged ethical concerns and conflict non-disclosure

This case study summarizes information from publicly available investigation reports, court records, and peer-reviewed publications, and discusses them in the context of research integrity scholarship.

At the end of the last century, University College London was considered one of the top UK institutions internationally. When the Shanghai Academic Ranking of World Universities commenced in 2003, it was ranked 20th. In 1998, an "early report" article from University College London was published in *The Lancet* after peer review. The journal publisher was Elsevier, which is reported to be one of the world's largest publishers of scientific, technical, and medical literature with over 2800 academic journals. *The Lancet* had a journal impact factor of around 12, and it ranked third in the Q1 quartile among journals in the general and internal medicine category in 1998. At that time, "early report" was a designated publication type in *The Lancet* intended for novel, preliminary, or hypothesis-generating findings that were considered important enough for rapid dissemination by the journal. The evidence presented in "early reports" was tentative rather than conclusive.

The 1998 *Lancet* paper was a case series of a dozen children, who the article said were "consecutively referred to the department." The paper was peer reviewed before publication and marked as an "early report" (Box 12.1). It explicitly stated that "investigations were approved by the Ethical Practices Committee … and parents gave informed consent." There were around one dozen co-authors from the same institution, University College London. No financial conflicts of interest were reported. The article suggested a link between exposure to the measles, mumps, and rubella (MMR) vaccination and autism. Within the evidence-based medicine hierarchy, a case series is the lowest form of evidence. In the absence of a controlled design, it would not have been possible to scientifically demonstrate causality. However, the lead author's press conference concerning the findings was covered in the mainstream media with much hype, and there emerged a trend of vaccine hesitancy in the public. In the UK, the MMR vaccination coverage started to decline (Box 12.2).

Shanghai ranking: Academic Ranking of World Universities, one of the most influential global research-based university rankings.

Impact factor: A journal statistic dividing the mean number of citations per article in a year by the total number of citable articles published in the previous two years.

Journal quartiles: A journal metric based on citation performance (e.g., impact factor, CiteScore, etc.) ranking all journals in a field into four equal groups, Q1–Q4.

Peer review: Evaluation of scientific manuscripts by others working in the same field, invited by journal editors before acceptance for publication as definitive articles representing the version of record.

The UK Legal Aid Board, now called the Legal Services Commission, had begun funding preliminary investigations for a multi-party litigation effort against MMR vaccine manufacturers. The lead author of the above paper had been recruited as an expert witness in 1996, according to reports. There was scientific evidence required to substantiate parental claims that the vaccine caused autism and bowel disorders in children. The board had approved an initial £55,000 grant for the lead author to conduct a study to establish causation for the lawsuits. The 1998 study was conducted with this initial grant administered through institutional accounts, and it was part of a broader strategy to build the legal case. However, as later reported, the co-authors of the paper or the editors of the journal in 1998 were unaware of the lead author's conflict of interest (the legal aid funding is said to have eventually totaled over £435,000, including fees and expenses to the lead author, according to reports). In the US, the 1998 paper was also cited in the early 2000s by claimants linking MMR to autism in the National Vaccine Injury Compensation Program in that country. The litigation grew to involve many claimants in both countries, but in the UK, the case collapsed in 2004.

A journalistic investigation revealed the Legal Aid grant and the failure to disclose this financial conflict in 2004. The allegations of misconduct led to an institutional inquiry at University College London. It identified a failure of declaration of conflicts of interest and stated that the work published had been "subjected to appropriate and rigorous ethical scrutiny." In the same issue where the institutional reply was published in *The Lancet* in 2004, a "retraction of an interpretation" appeared. It was issued by an author subgroup of a 1998 paper, not including the lead author. It stated that "in this paper no causal link was established" between the vaccine exposure and the outcome. The clarification amounted to an admission of reporting a conclusion more strongly worded than what was supportable by the study methodology, something that is described in the research integrity literature as spin or science hype (DOI: 10.1371/journal.pbio.2002173). There was no formal expression of concern issued by *The Lancet* at any stage.

Conflict of interest: Potential or perceived compromise in the objectivity or judgment of anyone involved in any aspect of research due to financial or personal (non-financial) interests. Failure of declaration is considered research misconduct.

Spin: Exaggerating the implications or importance of research findings.

Journalistic investigation: A systematic process of uncovering information on matters of public interest, such as research and publication integrity. It requires rigorous fact-checking usually involving multiple corroborating sources. Compared to general sleuthing, the work of journalists is governed by professional codes and regulations.

Box 12.1 Timeline of research integrity concerns: A case study of alleged ethical concerns and conflict non-disclosure in London

Dates	Brief overview of events
1996	**Lead author appointed as expert witness in a legal case and awarded a grant** The lead author of the paper in question became an expert in a legal case related to adverse effects of measles, mumps, and rubella (MMR) vaccination. He was awarded a grant of £55,000 by the UK Legal Aid Board for collating scientific evidence for the legal case. *Source: URLs: ethicsunwrapped.utexas.edu/case-study/birthing-vaccine-skepticism; centerforinquiry.org/wp-content/uploads/sites/33/quackwatch/gmc_findings.pdf.*
1998	**Article submission, peer review, and publication** An "early report" paper was published in *The Lancet* following peer review. The paper stated that "investigations were approved by the Ethical Practices Committee … and parents gave informed consent." No financial conflict of interest had been declared. The findings of the paper were widely covered in the mainstream media reportedly creating a scare about the MMR vaccination. *Source: DOI: 10.1016/s0140-6736(97)11096-0. URL: www.theguardian.com/society/2004/feb/24/publichealth.uknews.*
2004	**Allegations of research misconduct, informal institutional inquiry, and retraction of interpretation** A journalistic investigation in the *Sunday Times* newspaper reported that the lead author "did not tell his colleagues or medical authorities of this conflict of interest either during or after the research." Following an informal inquiry, the institution presented a clarification concerning the undisclosed conflict which appeared in *The Lancet* as a statement. The aspect concerning approval stated that the "wording in the published paper regarding Ethical Practice Committee approval and patient referral was accurate." At the same time, ten of the co-authors issued a formal retraction of interpretation in *The Lancet* stating that the in the 1998 paper "no causal link was established between MMR vaccine and autism as the data were insufficient." *Source: DOIs: 10.1016/S0140-6736(04)15699-7; 10.1016/S0140-6736(04)15715-2. URLs: briandeer.com/mmr/lancet-deer-1.htm; www.ucl.ac.uk/governance-compliance/sites/governance_compliance/files/mmr.pdf.*

2007–2010	**Professional regulator investigation and full article retraction** In a fitness to practice investigation undertaken over 200 days by the medical professional regulator of some of the co-authors, after a pre-hearing investigation there was a final disciplinary hearing. The findings showed failure to declare a conflict of interest as well as failure to obtain ethics committee approval. *The Lancet* retraction notice stated "that several elements of the 1998 paper … contrary to the findings of an earlier investigation. In particular, the claims in the original paper that children were 'consecutively referred' and that investigations were 'approved' by the local ethics committee have been proven to be false." *Source: DOI: 10.1016/S0140-6736(10)60175-4.*
2010	**Institutional response** Following the professional regulatory body's findings, the institution issued a statement that it had "learned a great deal from its involvement in the MMR issue and has now introduced a research governance framework that is robust and fit for purpose." *Source: URL: www.ucl.ac.uk/governance-compliance/sites/governance_compliance/files/mmr.pdf.*
2012	**Court judgment** The professional regulator's conclusion was challenged in court by one of the co-authors, not the lead author. The judge criticized the panel of the professional regulatory body in the published judgment. The independent medical practitioner tribunal service started the same year after this court judgment. *Sources: DOI: 10.1136/bmj.e1745; URL: bailii.org/ew/cases/EWHC/Admin/2012/503.html; pubpeer.com/publications/CF52AD098D3AC462697D50B97B3105.*

There were several papers involved; this chapter focuses on one paper, following it through in the timeline. See Box 12.2 for an outline of the research integrity roles of various actors in this case study and disclaimer.

Sources listed above are a few of the many that have covered this case study. This box summarizes reported allegations and findings; no judgment is intended.

Box 12.2 Retraction of an article and public health impact on the measles, mumps, and rubella (MMR) vaccination coverage

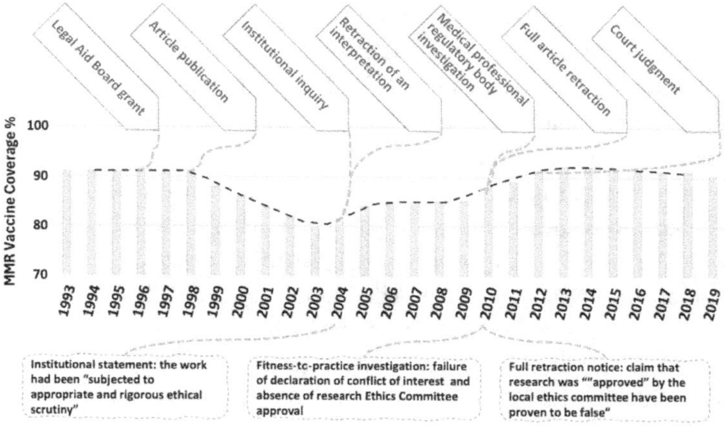

The above is a simplified description outlining the timing of investigations into allegations of research misconduct, article retraction, and the public health impact. The data are approximate; data sources include UK NHS Digital and UKHSA Childhood Vaccination Coverage Statistics.
See Box 12.1 for sources of information.
Adapted from: DOI: 10.1201/9781003655954.

The allegation of misconduct was also picked up by the doctors' professional regulatory body in the UK. A fitness to practice investigation of some medical co-authors, including the lead author, took place. Starting in 2007, the disciplinary hearing lasted over 200 days. It concluded in 2010, being one of the longest in the regulatory body's history. The findings were contained in a 143-page report. It agreed with the institutional inquiry on the failure to declare a conflict of interest. Importantly, it established that there had been no human research ethics committee approval. Moreover, it identified that the description of the participant sample as "consecutively referred" was not supported by the evidence. In 2010, *The Lancet* journal issued a full retraction, stating that claims made in the original paper regarding ethics approval and patient referral were inconsistent with findings reported in the professional regulatory investigation. Another article related to the 1998 *Lancet* "early report" published in the *American Journal of Gastroenterology*, authored by the research team at University College London, was also retracted based on the findings of the fitness to practice investigation (DOI: 10.1038/ajg.2010.149). The *European Journal of Gastroenterology & Hepatology* issued an expression of concern about a 2005 article by the same lead author that referred to the 1998 *Lancet* paper (DOI: 10.1097/MEG.0b013e328349d184). The fact that the institution and the professional regulator came to different conclusions on the status of the ethics committee approval

Expression of concern: A note published by a journal to inform readers of there being the possibility of a concern about the integrity of a paper.

Retraction: Removing a published paper from the research record due, for example, to the discovery of a flaw in its integrity.

was a key finding. According to the institution's own statements, it admitted that the 2004 inquiry was not a formal independent investigation.

In 2011, the *BMJ*, a London-based journal competing with The *Lancet*, published an article series authored by the investigative journalist who had initially reported the hidden funding behind the 1998 paper. He had now been able to compare the documents made public by the professional regulatory body's fitness to practice investigation with the findings reported in the 1998 article. There were misleading clinical descriptions in the published paper. The *BMJ* editorial associated with the article series covering the journalistic investigation claimed that there was "evidence of falsification of data" (DOI: 10.1136/bmj.c7452). Coincidentally, a correction to this editorial admitted the *BMJ* journal's own failure to declare financial conflict of interest on account of receiving "advertising and sponsorship revenue from vaccine manufacturers."

PubPeer: An online platform for post-publication peer review.

h(Hirsh)-index: A popular statistic to measure scientific output, taking account of citations, e.g., an *h*-index of 5 means that the author has 5 published papers that have been cited 5 times or more.

The professional regulatory body's outcome was challenged in court by one of the co-authors, not the lead author. The deliberations of the professional regulator were found to be inadequate in a 2012 court judgment. The court emphasized the need to differentiate between clinical care and research, and for clinical practitioners to avoid "undertaking research in the guise of clinical investigation and treatment." The 1998 paper remains retracted without any changes to the 2010 retraction notice. The court judgment was subsequently mentioned on PubPeer, which also linked the 1998 *Lancet* paper to the retraction and the expression of concern in other journals. The integrity issues covered by this case study relate to research ethics committee approval, failure of declaration of conflict of interest, the multiplicity of research misconduct investigations, and the retraction of an interpretation put forward in the original paper, followed by its full retraction.

Publicly available bibliometric indicator of the lead researcher's *h*-index could not be verified in 2025; the reasons for this were not publicly documented. The 1998 paper had been cited around 600 times till the partial retraction and around 1500 times in total before full retraction, according to Google Scholar. It has also been cited around 3000 times since the full retraction. A 2019 assessment of the citations had found that between 2005 and 2010, after the partial retraction, 38% of citations documented the retraction, while 72% did so after the full retraction (DOI:10.1001/jamanetworkopen.2019.15552). Only two journals issued a retraction or expression of concern about related publications (see above). University College London maintained its top ranking standing at 14th position in the Shanghai Academic

Ranking of World Universities in 2025 (Box 12.3). The recent *Lancet* journal impact factor was around 88, and it ranked first (Q1 quartile) among journals in the category of general and internal medicine, whereas it had ranked third in 1998. From a review of the journal archives, it appears that by the mid-2010s onward, the journal dropped the "early report" article type, and the current *Lancet* guidelines or instructions for authors do not mention it. This evolution reflects a move toward clearer labeling of research stages, ensuring preliminary work is not overstated. Changes in institutional rankings, article-level citations, academic indices, or journal metrics are reported descriptively only; no causal relationship with the case study is asserted or implied.

Box 12.3 Snapshot: The reported dimensions of research integrity issues in the case study of alleged ethical concerns and conflict non-disclosure in London

Actors and their research integrity roles (described without assessing adequacy or compliance with standards)	**Reported observations over case study timeline** (no causal inference implied)
Institution: University College London and its affiliated Royal Free Hospital	
• Responsible for overseeing research conduct of their staff. • Responsible for differentiating between clinical practice and research by training staff who have dual roles and giving oversight to the work. • Responsible for investigating allegations of research misconduct under its policies and procedures.	• A 1998 article retracted in 2010. • Finding of institutional inquiry refuted by professional regulatory investigation. • Journalistic investigation raised research integrity concerns. • Another related article retracted and one more expression of concern issued. • Introduced a revised institutional research governance framework post retraction. • University's Shanghai ranking increased.
Journal: *The Lancet*, published by Elsevier	

• Responsible for editorial assessment and peer review of submitted manuscripts before publication. • Responsible for timely engagement in post-publication integrity concerns raised under journal editorial policies.	• A 1998 article retracted fully in 2010 after a retraction of interpretation in 2004. • A related article retracted in another journal. • An expression of concern issued in another journal. • The journal impact factor increased, and quartile ranking was unchanged.
Funders:	
• Special Trustees of Royal Free Hampstead NHS Trust and the Children's Medical Charity named in the 1998 paper.	• No public comment noted.
Professional regulatory body and law courts	
• The UK General Medical Council (GMC) conducted a fitness to practice investigation.	• The GMC outcome was challenged in court, where it was criticized in the judgment.
Journalistic investigation	
• Journalistic investigation raised the integrity concerns that led to institutional inquiry and professional body investigation.	• Mainstream media and other medical journals covered the story.
UK Public Health Service	
• Measles, mumps, and rubella (MMR) vaccination program.	• A decline in vaccination coverage associated with measles outbreaks (Box 12.2).

See Box 1.1 for research integrity terminology.
See Box 1.2 for how research integrity concerns might arise and Box 1.3 for an outline of a research misconduct investigation.
See Box 12.1 for sources of information and the timeline of the case study.
Disclaimer: All factual statements are drawn from published literature and public records. No new allegation of research misconduct, dishonesty, or malice is intended or implied. The case study summarizes publicly available information and does not purport to determine liability or responsibility beyond what has been established in the cited records. References to individuals or organizations are made for academic discussion only and do not attribute intent or fault beyond the public record. When reporting changes in individual, institutional, organizational, and journal status or metrics, no causal inference is implied. The commentary and any opinions expressed are offered in good faith on matters of public interest concerning research integrity. Readers are encouraged to consult the original sources for full context.
University ranking data source: URL: www.shanghairanking.com/rankings/arwu/#### (year).
Journal impact factor and ranking are based on Journal Citation Reports.

Oversight via fitness to practice investigations

Drawing from the public records summarized above, the following analysis examines the role of professional regulatory bodies in addressing research misconduct and considers the broader public health implications of this case.

Analysis of this case study in terms of public health impact is important as the 1998 *Lancet* retracted article became pivotal to a UK MMR child vaccination controversy. Before its publication, MMR uptake exceeded 90% across the country. Following the paper's publication, MMR vaccination coverage declined in the UK during the early 2000s to approximately 80% (Box 12.2). Public health authorities and researchers have since associated this decline with increased vaccine hesitancy and subsequent measles outbreaks, including severe outcomes among some unvaccinated individuals. It was not until around 2015, following extensive public health education and recovery efforts, that MMR vaccination rates returned to their pre-1998 levels.

Investigations into allegations of research misconduct identified concerns relating to human research ethics committee approval and consent processes, and these issues could have been picked up by the journal had it asked for documentation on the first submission of the manuscript before its publication or at the time of investigation. The undisclosed financial conflict of interest (funding from legal sources linked to lawsuits against vaccine manufacturers) is attributed to inadequate disclosure by the lead author to editors and co-authors. There are established guidelines for the identification and management of conflicts of interest (Box 4.4). Professional regulatory body findings suggested selective patient recruitment and inaccuracies in reported clinical histories, which were characterized in subsequent commentaries as fabrication or falsification under research integrity frameworks. There also appeared to be an element of spin in writing conclusions in the original 1998 article, which was addressed by the 2004 partial retraction. After a journalistic investigation had raised concerns, the research integrity matters came under the purview of the medical professional regulatory body, as some of the co-authors were medical care providers to the children in the case series reported in the 1998 paper.

The regulatory body's responsibility extends to include research activities within the clinical practice of a doctor's work (Box 12.4). The codes of professional conduct require doctors to act with honesty, integrity, transparency, and respect for participants, principles that directly underpin research integrity. They are required to comply with the Declaration of Helsinki, a human research ethics document of the World Medical Association. When these standards are breached through inadequate ethical oversight, undisclosed conflicts of interest, data falsification, or selective reporting, regulators treat such failures as potential impairments of fitness to practice, thereby safeguarding both individual patients and broader public trust in health care. The retraction of the 1998 *Lancet* publication illustrates how regulatory oversight can become essential when research integrity in clinical care is questioned. The undisclosed financial interests tied to litigation against vaccine manufacturers became a trigger for the disciplinary hearing. Investigative journalism brought concerns to public attention, after which formal professional regulatory processes were initiated and concluded. The law court too became involved with the decision of the professional regulatory body, which was appealed.

Declaration of Helsinki: A living document on human research ethics produced and updated by the World Medical Association.

Accountability: A responsible research principle guiding individuals and organizations to be answerable for the research they engage in from idea to post-publication.

The case demonstrates how regulators bridge the gap between scientific publishing and doctors' professional accountability in the provision of healthcare. While journals handle post-publication corrections and institutions oversee research governance, regulatory bodies also enforce ethical and professional standards, ensuring that allegations of clinical research misconduct are addressed as a threat to patient and public safety. This example underscores the indispensable role of health profession regulators in the research ecosystem. By investigating and, where appropriate, sanctioning breaches of the code of conduct, regulators aim to deter future integrity concerns and reinforce public trust. The MMR controversy remains a powerful reminder that robust professional regulatory oversight is essential to prevent flawed research from undermining both individual health and societal well-being.

Box 12.4 An outline of fitness to practice investigations by professional regulatory bodies

Feature	Comments
Statutory purpose	Protect health, safety, and welfare of the public, ensuring standards in practice by establishing a code of conduct, licensing practitioners, and maintaining a register.
Code of conduct and research integrity	These codes emphasize evidence-based practice and engagement in research ethically and professionally to reduce uncertainty in evidence. Adhering to principles like human research ethics committee review, informed consent, and transparency, e.g., declaring conflicts of interest, are all part of the honesty and integrity required for ensuring standards.

Initial screening	Concerns may be raised by patients, employers, self-referral, police, or other sources, such as journalistic investigations. An initial inquiry undertakes screening or triage. If the matter raises a question of impaired fitness to practice, it proceeds to full investigation. If needed, an interim order, e.g., suspension or conditions, may be placed at this stage.
Investigation	Evidence, including medical records, witness statements, expert opinions, etc., are gathered, allegations are specified, and a response is sought from the practitioner. The case is reviewed by a panel. Unless there is closure without any further action, warnings may be issued, training may be required, or there may be referral to a fitness to practice panel if there is a prospect of proving impairment. The practitioner may appeal the outcome.
Fitness to practice hearing	This process is meant to be inquisitorial or truth-seeking rather than adversarial. Disciplinary hearing determines if the allegations are proven as facts (on balance of probabilities, not beyond reasonable doubt) and if there is impaired fitness to practice. If impaired, sanctions may be imposed, e.g., conditions, suspension, erasure from register. Decisions may be appealed in the court of law.
Research misconduct	Professional regulatory body and practitioners' employers may collaborate in investigation or share evidence. The facts established may be used by journals to retract published papers.

Policies and procedures vary by regulatory body; UK medical practitioners. URL: gmc-uk.org.

Chapter 12: Professional regulatory investigation: Alleged ethical failure and research misconduct in London – Key points

Advice for researchers

- Declare all conflicts of interest transparently, as undisclosed financial ties can lead to research misconduct allegations (Box 4.4).
- Make enhanced declarations; when in doubt, declare and share with co-authors and editors.
- Co-authors should actively verify findings reported (see Chapter 9).
- Ensure human research ethics committee approval and genuine participant informed consent (see also Chapters 4 and 10 concerning alleged ethical failures).

- Representing selectively recruited participants as "consecutive referrals" is widely regarded as inconsistent with research integrity standards.
- Describe the inclusion and exclusion criteria and the participant selection process accurately and in detail.
- Maintain data integrity; selective alteration of patient clinical histories has been classified in research integrity frameworks as fabrication or falsification.
- Take responsibility for carefully drafting the manuscript conclusions, avoiding spin when generating inferences from research findings; overclaiming causation may mislead readers and may require partial retraction.

Recommendations for journals and publishers

- Avoid obsession with novelty. Remove vague labels such as "early report" for classifying articles covering preliminary research findings. Stick to clear labels that correspond to established evidence-based medicine hierarchies.
- Concerning human research ethics committee approval and participant consent, a trust-based approach, i.e., a declaration in the text of the manuscript with availability of documents on request, is insufficient. Limiting requests for supporting documentation to cases of suspicion has been criticized as insufficient for ensuring publication integrity. For transparency, these documents should be routinely sought by journals and provided as supplementary materials for readers' reassurance (see also Chapters 4 and 10 concerning documentation of human research ethics committee approval as an integrity check).
- Strengthen pre-publication verification of conflicts; relying solely on author declarations is insufficient.
- Journals should transparently declare their own conflicts when publishing editorials (Box 4.4).
- Enhance transparency in peer review; publish comments and authors' responses with manuscripts published.
- Act swiftly on credible allegations; delays in retraction allow misinformation to spread. Deploy formal policies and procedures, instead of rapid informal inquiries as a knee-jerk reaction (Box 1.3).
- Publish reasons clearly in retraction notices.
- Deploy retraction of interpretations when spin has overinterpreted the findings of a study.

Roles of institutions and professional regulatory bodies

- The core mission of professional regulatory bodies to protect the public directly supports holding the profession accountable for research integrity when they engage in research; regulators can remove those from practice who seriously undermine trust through proven research misconduct (Box 12.4).

- Strengthen institutional oversight of research ethics and governance. Promote a culture of research integrity that does not tolerate research without human research ethics committee approval and informed consent (see Box 10.3 for an institutional action plan).
- Academic hospitals must ascertain that practitioners do not undertake research in the guise of clinical investigation and treatment.
- Implement clear policies on conflicts of interest and dual roles (Box 4.4).
- Institutions must require full disclosure of external funding, legal consulting roles, and any financial incentives at the outset of research. If funding is administered via institutional accounts, linkage to research approval and activity should be made explicit to identify gaps in compliance with research governance and the need for disclosure.
- Institutions should mandate regular research integrity training covering active involvement and accountability of co-authors (Box 7.1) and encourage reporting concerns without fear of retaliation for whistleblowing (Box 1.2).
- Institutions should enforce co-author responsibility, including ethics compliance, data verification, and accurate reporting. Co-author unawareness of the funding conflict raises suspicion about unethical authorship, also (see Chapter 9 for a case of alleged guest authorship).
- Conduct timely and thorough investigations when allegations arise, deploying formal policies and procedures (Box 1.3). Cooperate with other stakeholder organizations. Institutions must treat such cases as opportunities to refine policies, monitoring of clinician-researcher dual roles, audit processes, and communicate lessons to staff.

Glossary

This glossary uses information from the publications listed in the Suggested Reading section. The definitions provided here are those used in this book.

Academic Ranking of World Universities See **Shanghai Ranking.**

Accountability: A responsible research principle guiding individuals and organizations to be answerable for the research they engage in from idea to post-publication, including all aspects in the entire research lifecycle. It covers research approval, conduct, training, supervision, mentoring, publication, as well as societal impact (this is not a complete list). *Also see* **ALLEA**.

Adverse event: An undesirable and unintended harmful or unpleasant occurrence associated with an intervention. If there is a suggestion of a causal relationship, then the term used is adverse reaction. It may warrant prevention, specific treatment, alteration, or withdrawal of the intervention. *Also see* **Outcome adjudication committee**.

ALLEA: European Federation of Academies of Sciences and Humanities (ALL European Academies) is an independent body that advocates for the role of science as a global public good. It has issued a code for research integrity built upon four overarching principles, often summarized as the four I's: Reliability (ensuring the quality of research, reflected in the design, methodology, analysis, and use of resources); Honesty (developing, undertaking, reviewing, reporting, and communicating research in a transparent, fair, and unbiased way); Respect (for colleagues, research participants, society, ecosystems, cultural heritage, and the environment); and Accountability (for the research from idea to publication, and for its wider impacts) (allea.org). *Also see* **Research integrity** and **Accountability**.

AllTrials: A campaign for all past and present clinical trials to be registered and their methods and summary results reported (alltrials.net). *Also see* **Clinical trial**, **Randomized clinical trial**, and **RIAT**.

Applied research: Motivated by the desire to be useful in solving real-world problems, applied research aims to provide solutions. *Also see* **Basic research** and **Research translation**.

Artificial intelligence (AI): Automated solutions, using methods like machine learning, natural language processing, data mining, information retrieval, and other computer science methods to perform tasks that usually require human intelligence (language understanding, information retrieval, reasoning, learning, etc.). Traditional AI processes data to give results or predictions, e.g., plagiarism checks are automated. Unlike generative AI, traditional AI does not produce new content. *Also see* **Generative artificial intelligence (AI)**.

Audit: A planned formal evaluation of study conduct, i.e., activities, such as informed consent, and documents, such as data collection and recording, to independently determine if the study is being undertaken according to its approved protocol, and if it meets professional standards such as GCP or Good Clinical Practice in human clinical trials. *Also see* **Inspection, Forensic statistical analysis, GCP, Ethics**, and **Research governance**.

Authorship: Giving credit to those who design, conduct, analyze, and report a study, i.e., naming those who have made substantial contributions to the work leading to the completion of the study. Authors are accountable for the study in its published form. *Also see* **Authorship abuse**, **ICMJE**, and **CRediT**.

Authorship abuse: Authorship attribution that is not based strictly on contributions that meet authorship criteria. Authorship abuse occurs in many forms including: when authorship is demanded through coercion, e.g., based on seniority, rather than deserved on account of the contribution made (guest authorship); when someone is excluded from authorship even when they have made creditable contributions (ghost authorship); when someone is included as an author without their permission (invented authorship); when names of original contributors are removed in subsequent publications; when there is manipulation of the sequence of authors, particularly first, last, and corresponding author, without justification; etc. *Also see* **Guest authorship**.

Auto-plagiarism: *See* **Plagiarism**.

Balance of probabilities: Proving that something is more likely than not to have happened, i.e., over 50% probability. This is the standard of proof used in cases of research misconduct investigations. This is in sharp contrast to the "beyond reasonable doubt" yardstick applied in criminal cases in courts. Also note how vastly different the balance of probabilities rule is from the 95% probability threshold, $p<0.05$, used in scientific hypothesis testing.

Basic research: Motivated by curiosity, basic research aims to generate new knowledge. *Also see* **Applied research** and **Research translation**.

Bias (systematic error): A tendency for study results to depart systematically, either lower or higher, from the "true" results. Bias either exaggerates or underestimates the "true" effect of an intervention. Bias may arise due to systematic differences in comparison groups (selection bias), differences in care or exposure to factors other than the intervention of interest (performance bias), differences in assessment of outcomes (measurement bias), withdrawals or exclusions of participants enrolled in the study (attrition bias), etc. Studies with unbiased results are said to be internally valid. Bias is distinct from research integrity flaws that arise due to misconduct or questionable research practices. *Also see* **Validity (internal validity)** and **Random error**.

Breach of contract: A legal cause of action in which a binding agreement, e.g., in an academic-industry partnership, is not honored by one or more of the parties through nonperformance or interference with the other party's performance.

Case report form: A paper-based or electronic document used for data collection from each consenting participant enrolled in clinical research. The forms contain the research data in raw form. Once collected, the data are entered into a database and used for statistical analysis and reporting. The protection of participant privacy and confidentiality is a key issue in data collection and processing. Where case report forms are shared with a regulator of drugs and devices, they are often redacted to deidentify or anonymize them. *Also see* **Clinical trial**, **GCP**, **Audit**, and **Research governance**.

Cherry-picking: Reporting particular data and results while omitting others. *Also see* **p-hacking**.

Citation: A reference to the original source of information written in an article, such as an idea, claim, quote, figure, method, or any other aspect of the writing that is not the author's own. Citations protect intellectual property, giving credit to the original author, and allow readers to find the source and evaluate it themselves if they so wish. Citations are used to avoid plagiarism, support the claims made with evidence, and demonstrate how the article has been informed by other works. Citations should be relevant, complete, and accurate in order for bibliometric analyses and indices, such as *h*-index, impact factor, CiteScore, etc., to serve as valid measures of academic performance. *Also see* **Citation, h(Hirsh)-index, Impact factor, CiteScore, Inadequate citation practices**, and **Publication process manipulation**.

Citation concentration index (c^2-index): Citation manipulation often has its origin in a few sources. c^2-index aims to quantify this. It is a number N where there are N citing papers that each cite the researcher at least N times (and the remaining citing papers cite them fewer than N times). High c^2 values indicate concentrated citations from a few sources, potentially signaling manipulation (DOI: 10.1038/s41598-025-88709-7). *Also see* **Citation, Inadequate citation practices**, and **Publication process manipulation**.

CiteScore: A journal metric that calculates the average number of citations received per document published (articles, reviews, conference papers, etc.) in a four-year period. It is calculated using citation data from the Scopus database. *Also see* **Scopus, Citation**, and **Impact factor**.

Clinical study report: A report prepared in a highly structured format presented to a drug or device regulator in the form of an information dossier about the planning, execution, results, and analysis of a clinical trial. *Also see* **Regulator of drugs and devices**.

Clinical trial: In the biomedical literature, it is a loosely defined term generally meaning a study of the effects of healthcare interventions. The term encompasses a range of study designs, including large randomized clinical trials of patients at one end and uncontrolled observations of a few healthy volunteers at the other. Clinical trials are conducted in phases for drug regulatory approval. Phase I clinical trial focuses on the safety of an intervention in a few healthy human volunteers; randomization is not used. Phase II clinical trial gathers preliminary evidence on whether an intervention works in human participants. It may or may not involve randomization. The preliminary evidence gathered may be used to help define the intervention better, including dose finding (Phase IIa) studies, and efficacy studies with a randomized clinical trial in a small number of carefully selected participants with the disease or condition targeted by the intervention (Phase IIb). Phase III clinical trial gathers evidence on the effectiveness of an intervention. Also called a confirmatory trial, it involves randomization of a large number of human participants with the disease or condition targeted by the intervention. Prevention trials, such as vaccine trials, recruit healthy participants. Phase IV clinical trial gathers additional information about an approved drug's safety or optimal use in healthcare practice. *Also see* **Randomized clinical**

trial and **Effectiveness**.

CoARA: The Coalition for Advancing Research Assessment commits to reviewing and developing criteria, tools, and processes for assessing research organizations, and to abandoning inappropriate uses of quantitative journal- and publication-based metrics (coara.org). *Also see* **Publish or perish**, **SCOPE**, and **DORA**.

Coercive citation practices: Peer reviewers and journals may coerce authors into including references to their own papers during manuscript revisions to boost their own citation metrics, such as *h*-index and impact factor. Senior academics in a position of power may coerce colleagues and junior academics into citing their works in manuscripts, whether or not they are co-authors. *Also see* **Citation**, **h(Hirsh)-index**, **Impact factor**, **CiteScore**, **Inadequate citation practices**, and **Publication process manipulation**.

Colonization of research: A systemic mindset and power structure that perpetuates historical colonial hierarchies in Global North–South research partnerships, where researchers from high-income countries dominate agenda-setting, knowledge production, and benefit accrual, treating low- and middle-income countries as objects of study rather than equal partners. *Also see* **Ethics**, **Ethics dumping**, **Parachute research**, and **Power**.

Complainant: *See* **Whistleblower**.

Complaint: A written notification of a suspected case of research misconduct or questionable research practice made to a body that has an investigative role, e.g., institution, funder, journal, professional regulatory body, etc. The notification is sometimes also known as a formal complaint. Complaints can be lodged anonymously. *Also see* **GCP**, **Questionable research practice**, **Research integrity**, and **Research misconduct**.

Composite outcome: Combination of two or more component outcomes into a composite. Participants may be said to have experienced the composite outcome when they suffer any one of the components. Composite outcomes are used when individual core outcomes have low event rates. In this situation, composite outcomes can be constructed to help reduce the sample size or the follow-up period or both to make for a feasible study. The components of the composite outcome should be of a similar level of patient relevance, similar frequency of occurrence over the follow-up period, and similar in response to the intervention. Otherwise, it may be difficult to interpret effects comparing composite outcomes between groups. *Also see* **Outcome** and **Effect**.

Confidentiality: Keeping disclosed information private. In research misconduct investigations, organizations and individuals involved have an obligation to keep the information shared with them under their own control. Disclosure is made only on a need-to-know basis. Confidentiality breach is a form of research misconduct whereby organizations and individuals make unauthorized disclosures to others concerning information shared with them in confidence. Explicit prior permission is required from the owner of the information for proper disclosure. In some circumstances, disclosure may be required by law. *Also see* **Defamation** and **Research misconduct**.

Confidentiality breach: *See* **Confidentiality**.

Conflict of interest: Potential or perceived compromise in the objectivity or judgment of anyone involved in research and publication (research supervisor, author, editor, peer reviewer, human research ethics committee member, funding panel member, study oversight committee member, research misconduct investigation committee member, etc.) due to financial or personal (non-financial) interests. Financial interests include anything where payment is involved, e.g., employment, research and project funding, consultancies, ownership of stock and shares or options, honoraria, patents, paid expert testimony, etc. A distinction is made between funding directly supporting a particular research project and that obtained for other projects. Personal interests that could influence objectivity or judgment are harder to identify and may include academic rivalries, intellectual passions, religious or political beliefs, etc. The existence of a conflict of interest does not automatically mean that there is or has been a compromise; transparency requires declaration. Lack of declaration of conflicts of interest is research misconduct. ICMJE provides a proforma for this declaration (icmje.org/disclosure-of-interest). *Also see* **Funding disclosure** and **Research misconduct**.

COPE: Committee on Publication Ethics. Among other things, it issues guidance to journals on handling allegations of research misconduct (publicationethics.org). *Also see* **Journal**, **ICMJE**, and **WAME**.

Corresponding author: An author of a paper who is responsible for communication with the journal during the manuscript submission, its peer review, revisions, and publications, and subsequently in any post-publication correspondence. Corresponding status is considered a prestigious authorship role. *Also see* **Authorship**.

Corrigendum: The publication of a correction notice concerning a paper's version of record. A corrigendum refers to the correction of an author's error(s) in the research work where some elements of the paper may be affected, but its research integrity and main findings remain intact. A corrigendum requires approval by the authors and may be subject to editorial and peer review assessment. By contrast, an erratum, also a correction notice, refers to a journal's error in the publishing process, and it may be issued by the journal. *Also see* **Version of record**, **Retraction**, **Research misconduct**, and **Erratum**.

CRediT: Contributor Roles Taxonomy is a system for classifying the roles played by individual authors and those acknowledged in a publication. It recognizes and defines the following contributions (in alphabetical order): conceptualization (structured question formulation or development of research goals, aims, objectives, hypothesis, etc.); data curation (data annotation, producing metadata necessary for interpreting the data itself, and maintaining research data for initial use and later reuse); formal analysis (applying statistical, mathematical, computational, or other formal techniques to analyze or synthesize data); funding acquisition (obtaining financial support for the study leading to this publication); investigation (conducting a study according to its approved protocol including data collection); methodology (designing a study); project administration (managing, coordinating, and executing a study); resources (providing study materials, computing resources, etc.); review and editing of draft (critical reviewing, commenting on, or revising the initial manuscript draft); software (programming, software development, designing computer programs, implementation of the computer code and supporting algorithms, etc.); supervision (oversight and leadership responsibility for research planning and execution, including mentorship); validation (replication or reproducibility of results); visualization (preparing data presentation); and writing of original draft (preparing the initial draft of the manuscript to be submitted for publication) (DOI: 10.1087/20150211). *Also see* **Funding disclosure** and **Authorship abuse**.

Data sharing: The data transparency principle that studies should share the deidentified or anonymized dataset to allow independent replication of the reported results as well as to derive other benefits such as contribution to evidence syntheses with individual participant data (IPD) meta-analyses and performance of secondary analyses. This requires sharing the full analyzable dataset derived from the raw data accompanied by metadata describing the dataset. It should be prepared deidentified in compliance with privacy laws and sited in a secure repository. Data sharing acronym FAIR abbreviates that data should be Findable, Accessible, Interoperable, and Reusable (DOI: 10.1038/sdata.2016.18). *Also see* **Individual participant data (IPD) meta-analyses**.

Data sleuthing: *See* **Sleuthing**.

Declaration of Helsinki: *See* **Helsinki declaration**.

Defamation: Discrediting someone or harming their reputation through a false verbal, video (slander), or written (libel) communication. Confidentiality is required in whistleblowing and research misconduct investigations to help protect against causing defamation. Making a statement (which turns out to be false) in good faith during the course of a duty, such as reporting suspected misconduct to the research integrity office, is not defamation. Such a statement should not be made with malice, i.e., with knowledge that it is false or with reckless disregard for whether it is true or not, and it should not be shared with those who do not need to know. *Also see* **Whistleblower** and **Confidentiality**.

DORA: The Declaration on Research Assessment (DORA) recognizes the need to improve how researchers and their outputs are evaluated, eliminating the use of journal-based metrics, and instead assessing research on its own merits, in funding, appointment, and promotion considerations (sfdora.org). *Also see* **Publish or perish**, **SCOPE**, and **CoARA**.

Duplication: *See* **Plagiarism**.

Effectiveness : The extent to which an intervention produces a beneficial effect in the routine setting. Efficacy is the extent to which an intervention can produce a beneficial effect in an ideal, highly controlled setting. Unlike efficacy, effectiveness seeks to address the question: does an intervention work under ordinary day-to-day circumstances? *Also see* **Clinical trial**.

Erratum: The publication of a correction notice concerning a paper's version of record. The term erratum refers to the correction of a journal's error in the publishing process. A minor publishing error may be corrected by the journal without any author input, but authors should be notified. *Also see* **Version of record**, **Retraction**, **Corrigendum**, and **Research misconduct**.

Ethics: Decision-making guided by moral values that distinguish between right and wrong. The fundamental ethical principles are beneficence (promote well-being), non-maleficence (not harm), autonomy (self-determination), and justice (fairness). *Beneficence* is the fundamental research ethics principle that research ought to be undertaken for societal benefit. Benefits may also arise for participants through the process of taking part in research, and this ought to be balanced against the potential risks. *Non-maleficence* is the fundamental research ethics principle that potential risks to participants ought to be balanced against the benefits to be gained from undertaking research. The monitoring of risks to participants is a key obligation on the part of researchers and institutional research governance offices. Depending on the level of risk, independent data monitoring committees may be required to protect participants. *Autonomy* is the fundamental research ethics principle that potential participants should make their own independent, informed, and entirely voluntary decision to sign up for research. *Justice* is the fundamental research ethics principle of fairness. To meet this principle, research must address a relevant societal priority, its participants ought to come from the same population that is expected to reap the benefits of the findings of the completed research, exclusion criteria cannot unjustifiably be based on a particular characteristic protected by law, etc. *Also see* **Moral values** and **Human research ethics committee**.

Ethics dumping: Exploitative practices in research partnerships involving high-income and low-income settings whereby the high-income partner takes advantage of the imbalances of power, resources, and knowledge. The global code of conduct for equitable research partnerships, also known as the TRUST code, stipulates the inclusion of lower-income settings throughout the research and publication process (globalcodeofconduct.org). *Also see* **Ethics**, **Parachute research**, **Colonization of research**, and **Power**.

Evidence-based medicine (EBM): Also known as evidence-based practice (EBP), it is the conscientious, explicit, and judicious use of current best research evidence in making healthcare decisions. It involves the process of systematically finding, appraising, and using contemporaneous research findings as the basis for clinical decisions. Another related term, evidence-based healthcare, extends EBM to all professions associated with healthcare, including purchasing and management. EBM evidence validity hierarchy places randomized evidence at the top, while case reports and uncontrolled case series are at the bottom. *Also see* **Randomized clinical trial** and **Systematic review**.

Expression of concern: A note published by a journal to inform readers of there being the possibility of a concern about the integrity of a paper. *Also see* **Retraction**, **Research misconduct**, and **Questionable research practices**.

Fabrication: Making up data or results for using them as if they were genuine. It is one of the three cardinal sins listed in the FFP definition of research misconduct. *Also see* **FFP**, **Questionable research practices**, and **Research misconduct**.

False Claims Act: All countries have laws designed to combat fraud against the government. In the United States, this is called the False Claims Act. These laws prohibit individuals or companies from knowingly submitting false or fraudulent claims for payment to the federal government, or causing such claims to be submitted. Failing to disclose known research integrity issues (like research misconduct concerns) in federal research grant applications can fall under the jurisdiction of these laws if the proposals submitted are shown to rely on inaccurate or incomplete information. In the United States, whistleblowers who file lawsuits on behalf of the government can receive a share of any recovery. *See* **Sleuthing**.

Falsification: Manipulating or omitting research data or results and using them as if they were genuine. For example, a data subset that does not support a desired conclusion may be omitted. Image manipulation is also a form of falsification. It is one of the three cardinal sins listed in the FFP definition of research misconduct. *Also see* **FFP**, **Questionable research practices**, and **Research misconduct**.

FFP: Fabrication, Falsification, and Plagiarism, regarded as the unholy trinity or the cardinal sins that define research misconduct. There are many other practices included in the definition of research misconduct depending on the jurisdiction. *Also see* **Questionable research practices** and **Research misconduct**.

Fishing expedition: Performing multiple tests in a dataset without an *a priori* hypothesis and statistical analysis plan. For instance, repeatedly categorizing continuous variables without justification until a particular cut-off gives a statistically significant result. *Also see* **p-hacking**, **Selective outcome reporting**, and **Statistical analysis plan**.

For Better Science: A crowd-sourced project running a website with the help of an international team of research integrity experts (forbetterscience.com). *Also see* **Sleuthing**.

Forensic statistical analysis: An analysis undertaken in the investigation of alleged research misconduct. Using the dataset of the study that is the subject of the allegation, forensic statistics are applied to check the raw data file, the statistical analysis file derived from the raw dataset or the statistical analyses reported, etc. The raw data examination may include checks for data ranges, distributions, digit preference, etc. There may be a need to revert to the original case report forms to ensure that the dataset includes the data actually collected. *Also see* **Case report form** and **Research misconduct**.

Fraud: Any intentional act of deception in research violating research integrity. *Also see* **Research misconduct**.

Funder: An organization that provides funding for undertaking a study. The funders may be government agencies, philanthropists, research charities, industry (e.g., pharmaceutical and medical device) companies, etc. Funders may provide money through grants or donations given to institutions administered through contractual agreements. The main funder has a role in scientific quality assurance and securing value for money. *Also see* **Funding disclosure**, **Funding effect Journal**, and **Institution**.

Funding disclosure: A section of the protocol, article, conference abstract, etc. describing the funding directly supporting the research being presented. In article submission, this disclosure is usually added in the journal's online portal. It should include the specific grant numbers and full names of funders. Funders themselves may stipulate how their support should be stated. The disclosure must be specific to the research being reported. Beware that omitting a funder, even if in error, may be perceived as an attempt to hide the support provided. The manuscript should state if the funder played any role in the study design, conduct, analysis, and reporting. This disclosure is in addition to declaring conflicts of interest. *Also see* **Conflict of interest**, **Funder**, and **Research misconduct**.

Funding effect: The pressure to prove a specific hypothesis linked to funding. Funding effect specifically occurs when the pressure comes from a secondary interest (financial or contractual) associated with funding, which compromises the primary interest of the scientific truth. The researcher's objectivity is challenged by the pressure to deliver a pre-determined outcome considered desirable by a funder. If the hypothesis is linked to the business interest of a drug or device company, then sometimes the term financial sponsorship bias is used. The term hypothesis pressure, also called confirmation bias or investigator bias, may be used to refer to the academic pressure to prove one's own theory to gain prestige or grants for career advancement. *Also see* **Funder** and **Funding disclosure**.

GCP: Good clinical practice in human clinical trials or GCP is a set of internationally recognized ethical and professional standards for the design, conduct, recording, analysis, and reporting of human clinical research. In some jurisdictions, researchers are required to have GCP certification updated every two years. *Also see* **Research integrity** and **Standard**.

Generative artificial intelligence (AI): Artificial Intelligence or AI developments within computer sciences, e.g., ChatGPT or Generative Pretrained Transformer, based on large language models. It goes a step further than traditional AI in that it generates or produces new content, such as text, graphs, images, etc. It can be deployed in manuscript writing, peer review, and editing, among many other possibilities. Regarding its use, transparency is required in the publication process. This book uses various generative AI tools for searching and summarizing literature. *Also see* **Artificial intelligence (AI)**.

Gift authorship: *See* **Guest authorship**.

Good faith: Acting with honesty, sincerity, and fairness, without the intent to deceive, defraud, or take unfair advantage. *Also see* **Whistleblower**.

Good publication practice: Publication practice that is compliant with ethical and professional principles and standards. GPP is an abbreviation for professional guidance on medical writing for the publication of commercially sponsored biomedical research, be it in the form of manuscripts, conference abstracts, or posters, etc. (DOI: 10.7326/M15-0288). *Also see* **Research integrity**.

Good Research Practice: *See* **GCP**.

Good Scientific Practice: *See* **GCP**.

Google Scholar: A freely accessible web search engine that indexes the full text or metadata of scholarly literature across a wide range of publishing formats and disciplines, aggregating from nearly all major publishers, universities, preprint repositories, and specialized scholarly sources, i.e., almost any work that has a DOI. As a broad and inclusive index, it captures conference abstracts and proceedings that might be excluded by more selective databases like Web of Science and Scopus. It calculates and displays metrics such as the *h*-index, which includes self-citations. Some databases, like Web of Science and Scopus, offer options to view citation metrics excluding self-citations. *Also see* ***h*-index**, **Scopus**, and **Web of Science**.

GPP: *See* **Good Publication Practice**.

Guest authorship: Listing those people as co-authors who have not made substantial contributions. Synonyms include courtesy, gift, and honorary authorship. Gift authorship is often offered or sought in the context of supervision and mentorship, or as a goodwill gesture in advance of a future research collaboration. Coercion authorship involves bullying the junior research team members or students into delivering a gift authorship to the supervisor. The ICMJE criteria are relevant for defining a level contribution that merits authorship. *Also see* **Authorship abuse** and **Authorship**.

Guideline: Also known as clinical practice guideline, it is a collation of statements that aim to assist practitioners and patients in making decisions about specific clinical situations. Guidelines often, but not always, deploy evidence syntheses, e.g., in the form of systematic reviews. *Also see* **Systematic review**.

h(Hirsh)-index: A statistic to measure scientific performance, taking account of citations. It is frequently used by institutions in appointments, appraisals, and promotions of academic staff and by funders in research grant assessments and awards. For a researcher, it is calculated by placing papers co-authored by them in rank order of citations (including self-citation in some databases), and the value *h* is the number of the rank that is the same as the number of citations. So, an *h*-index of 5 means that the author has 5 published papers that have been cited 5 times or more. Authors may, e.g., through a combination of collaboration authorship, guest authorship, coercive citation practices, and gratuitous citations (influencing colleagues to cite them), be able to manipulate this index. It appears that the *h*-index calculation makes no adjustments for article retraction. The *h*-index produced by the Scopus database tends to be intermediate between that obtained via Web of Science and Google Scholar. On average, across all disciplines and subjects hypothetically, if the *h*-index for early career researchers is 5–10, that for independent researchers at assistant professor and lecturer level, it could be 10–15, for established researchers at associate professor level, it could be 15–30, for full professors it could be above 30, and for field leaders it could be above 60. Discipline- and subject-specific ranges and comparisons are more appropriate. Journals may also be evaluated using the *h*-index in addition to the impact factor. Coercive citation practices may be deployed by peer reviewers and journals to manipulate these indices. *Also see* **Citation**, **Coercive citation practices**, **Inadequate**

citation practices, **Scopus**, **Web of Science**, **Google Scholar**, **Impact factor**, **CiteScore**, and **Publication process manipulation**.

Halo effect: Highly prolific or renowned researchers, e.g., Nobel laureates, may be subjected to less scrutiny by journals, peer reviewers, and data sleuths. However, they have earned retractions of their articles, so there is no place for double standards in research integrity assessments. The same phenomenon applies to highly profile institutions and journals. *Also see* **Publication asymmetry**.

Helsinki Declaration: The Declaration of Helsinki is widely considered the cornerstone of human research ethics. Produced by the World Medical Association (WMA) first in 1964, it is a living document periodically revised, outlining and updating ethical principles for medical research involving human participants. *Also see* **Ethics** and **Human research ethics committee**.

Highly prolific authorship: Defined as authors who publish one full paper every five days (more than 72 full papers annually). It may be achieved without meeting authorship criteria, particularly the criterion concerning approval of the manuscript (DOI: 10.1038/d41586-018-06185-8). In this case, it may become a form of guest authorship. *Also see* **Authorship abuse** and **Guest authorship**.

Human research ethics committee : Known also by acronyms like REC (Research Ethics Committee) or IRB (Institutional Review Board), these committees are set up under national research regulatory laws. Their membership, including lay members, should have the expertise required to assess the ethical issues in studies. They are tasked principally with the responsibility of giving formal approval to a study proposal and monitoring the ethical conduct of the studies approved (in some settings, the compliance monitoring role may be undertaken by research governance offices set up by institutions). They may also engage in the education and training of researchers. Note that human research ethics committees are different from ethics committees in hospitals and clinics that address questions related to clinical care. *Also see* **Ethics** and **Research governance**.

ICMJE: International Committee of Medical Journal Editors. Among other things, it defines the criteria for authorship and gives other guidance such as registration of clinical trials (icmje.org). *Also see* **WAME** and **COPE**.

Impact factor (Journal Impact Factor): A popular statistic for ranking journals in order of perceived importance. It is calculated as the mean number of citations per article in a year, with the denominator being the total number of citable articles published in the previous two years in a given journal. *Trials*, an open-access journal that charges article processing fees and covers all aspects of randomized clinical trials in healthcare, had a 2022 impact factor of 2.5, i.e., the citable articles it published in 2020 and 2021 were cited on average 2.5 times in 2022 (including self-citation). There are variations on this approach deployed to create different indices, e.g., CiteScore, five-year impact factor, and others. Journals may deploy coercive citation practices to manipulate these indices. Retracted articles are included in the denominator, but citations to retracted articles are excluded from the numerator. This means retractions can lower the impact factor. *Also see* **Citation**,

CiteScore, Coercive citation practices, Inadequate citation practices, and **Publication process manipulation.**

Inadequate citation practices: Erroneously included citations in published articles. These may include unnecessary self-citation as well as citations of works of others that are inappropriate, irrelevant, misleading, missing, inaccurate, etc. Authors should only cite relevant works after reading the full text and without any coercion or pressure. *Also see* **Citation, CiteScore, Questionable research practices,** and **Coercive citation practices.**

Initial public offering (IPO): The first time that a private company sells shares of its stock to the public on a stock exchange. It raises significant capital for growth or paying down debt that the company might have accrued as a spinout. Company founders, early backers, and employees can realize gains on their investments through an IPO. *Also see* **Security.**

Inspection: An audit of a research study conducted by an external, legally competent authority, such as a drug or device regulator. It has serious implications for the researchers and their institutions in case of a finding of noncompliance with professional standards such as GCP or Good Clinical Practice in human clinical trials. *Also see* **Audit, GCP, Ethics,** and **Research governance.**

Institution: A clinical academic organization, e.g., a university or a hospital, that employs researchers. The institution's role covers the lifecycle of a study leading up to its publication, and it focuses on research ethics and governance; journals focus on communication. Funders offer institutions money to support studies under contractual agreements. Institutions tend to have their own research integrity policies and misconduct investigation procedures, which may operate under the umbrella of national research integrity laws in some countries. *Also see* **Research governance, Ethics, Sponsor, Journal,** and **Funder.**

Institutional Review Board (IRB): *See* **Human Research Ethics Committee.**

Intellectual honesty: An honest attitude in the pursuit of truth. In research, this may be demonstrated through the acknowledgment of original sources for the ideas used to generate the hypotheses tested, the presentation of facts in an unbiased manner devoid of spin that gives an unjustifiable positive impression in manuscripts, the avoidance of plagiarism, etc. Note that honest errors do not constitute intellectual dishonesty or research misconduct. *Also see* **Scientific virtue, Research integrity,** and **Research misconduct.**

Intervention: A therapeutic or preventative regimen, e.g., a drug, an operative procedure, a dietary supplement, an educational leaflet, a test (followed by a treatment), a mobile health application, etc., undertaken with the aim of improving health outcomes. *Also see.*

IPO: *See* **Initial public offering (IPO).**

JIF: *See* **Impact factor.**

Journal: An establishment composed of editors and other publishing staff who organize peer review of study manuscripts submitted by authors, and publishes digital or print (paper-based) versions of the accepted scientific papers. Journals operate during the study lifecycle, focusing on the communication of information, e.g., they publish protocols during the early life of a study and findings after the study is completed. *Also see* **Open access publication**, **WAME**, **ICMJE**, and **COPE**.

Journal Impact Factor: *See* **Impact factor**.

Journal quartiles (Q1: -Q4) A journal metric based on citation performance (impact factor, CiteScore, etc.) ranking all journals in a field into four equal groups: Q1 or top 25% are considered top-performing; Q2 or 25–50% are above-average; Q3 or 50–75% are below-average; and Q4 or bottom 25% are the lowest-ranking. *Also see* **CiteScore** and **Impact Factor**.

Journalistic investigation: Investigative journalism is a systematic process of uncovering information that is either hidden or difficult to access, often involving matters of public interest such as research and publication integrity. It requires rigorous fact-checking, usually involving multiple corroborating sources, before the publication of the news story. Compared to sleuthing, the work of journalists is governed by professional codes and regulations. *See* **Sleuthing**.

Liquidation: The process of ending a business and distributing its remaining assets due to insolvency or an inability to repay its debts.

Market capitalization: The value of a public company traded on the stock market, calculated by multiplying the total number of shares by the share price. *Also see* **Security**.

Misconduct: *See* **Research misconduct**.

Misrepresentation: Also known as misquotation, it is the incorrect or misleading use of another author's words or ideas in a way that distorts their original meaning. *Also see* **Plagiarism**.

Moral values: A set of principles that differentiate right from wrong. *Also see* **Ethics**, **Principle**, and **Standard**.

Need to-know: A confidentiality standard used by organizations to limit the flow of sensitive information. *Also see* **Confidentiality**.

Open access publication: Open knowledge dissemination via free of cost, immediate availability of research outputs and articles online including journal articles. It comes in many forms. At the top end, there is immediate open access to the version of record of the article that comes all singing, all dancing as published formally by the journal (gold open access). The other options include preprints or accepted manuscripts before copyediting self-archived by authors, possibly with an embargo period introducing some delay in open access (green open access). The future may see the development of legitimate academic-led publishing initiatives that offer immediate open access totally free (diamond open access). *Also see* **Open science**, **Version of record**, and **Journal**.

Open peer review: An umbrella term for the various options available to make peer review compatible with open science principles, including naming peer reviewers (open identities), publishing peer review reports and authors' responses alongside articles (open reports, ideally with DOIs assigned), enabling wider participation in the review process, e.g., by making preprints immediately available on submission for public comment (open pre-review), etc. *Also see* **Open science**, **PubPeer**, and **Peer review**.

Open science: An umbrella term covering various initiatives like prospective public research registration, open peer review, open access publications, open research data, citizen science, etc. that encourage sharing, cooperation, and knowledge dissemination without restrictions. Citizen science encourages public and consumer involvement in scientific research, with citizens actively making intellectual contributions, not simply participating passively as research subjects. Lay members of the public may give input in areas such as priority setting, core outcome selection, protocol development, consent procedures, participant recruitment and retention, etc. Thus, citizen science is research being carried out with or by citizens rather than it being undertaken about or for them. *Also see* **Research transparency**.

OpenAlex: Named after the library of Alexandria in Egypt, it is an open-access bibliographic catalogue of research articles, authors, and institutions (https://openalex.org).

Organization: Any entity, be it an institution, funder, university, hospital, publisher, any regulator, etc., that is a legally constituted body to undertake a function. With this role comes organizational responsibility, e.g., establishing a workplace culture. The personal responsibility individual organizational employees or members have is distinct from the organizational responsibilities that come with their role as legal entities. *Also see* **Institution**, **Funder**, and **Journal**.

Outcome: The changes in health status that arise from the disease or condition targeted by interventions or exposure. The intervention aims to reduce bad outcomes (e.g., mortality in cancer) or increase good outcomes (e.g., pregnancy in infertility). Subjective outcomes may require the input of an outcome adjudication committee blind to participants' group allocation to reduce the risk of measurement bias. The comparison of outcomes between groups is used to estimate the effect of interventions. *Also see* **Composite outcome**, **Effect**, and **Outcome adjudication committee**.

Outcome adjudication committee: Outcomes, including adverse events, may be best adjudicated by independent experts or researchers blind to participants' group allocation. This approach aims to standardize outcome assessment against protocol-specified criteria, minimizing the risk of measurement bias in studies with subjectivity in assessments. *Also see* **Adverse event**, **Outcome**, and **Measurement bias**.

p-hacking: A manipulation of data analysis whereby different statistical tests are repeatedly applied until one of them turns up significant, i.e., the p-value observed crosses the statistical significance threshold (e.g., $p<0.05$). To avoid this problem, an *a priori* statistical analysis plan should pre-specify a single analytic strategy for testing the main hypothesis concerning the primary outcome. Harking is another related term similar to cherry-picking, fishing expedition, and p-hacking. This term refers to hypothesizing with the benefit of hindsight, i.e., after the results of multiple tests in a dataset are known. *Also see* **p-value**, **Statistical analysis plan**, and **Selective outcome reporting**.

Parachute research: Exploitative practices where researchers from high-income settings collect data and samples from lower-income settings, without meaningful local involvement or collaboration, often neglecting local knowledge and failing to address local needs. Other synonymous terms used to describe these exploitative or colonial practices include helicopter research, annexed sites, and postal research. *Also see* **Ethics**, **Ethics dumping**, **Colonization of research**, and **Power**.

Participants: Individuals, also known as subjects, who meet the eligibility criteria and give informed consent for taking part in a research study. Study interventions target the disease or condition participants have. After human research ethics committee approval, eligible and consenting participants are included in a study and followed up until outcome data are collected. Participation is voluntary and guided by informed consent. Healthcare professionals are responsible for ensuring that patients are not forced to enter into studies. *Also see* **Intervention** and **Outcome**.

Peer review: Formal evaluation of a scientific manuscript by others working in the same field before its publication as a definitive article representing the version of record. Traditionally, peer review is undertaken at the invitation of journal editors with the objective of having the submitted manuscripts assessed for their merit, including, among other things, a filter for research integrity and quality. The traditional peer review is single-blind in that the identity of the peer reviewer is kept concealed from the authors, something that impinges on accountability and transparency. Pre-review and post-publication peer review are uninvited evaluations, and authors have a duty to respond to all the comments made, whether or not formally invited by the journal. *Also see* **Sleuthing**, **Accountability**, **PubPeer**, and **Open peer review**.

Plagiarism: Copying the work of others (text, tables, images, data, etc.) and presenting it as if it were one's own work without proper citation to the original source. The Latin root of the word, *plagium*, means kidnapping. Self-plagiarism, auto-plagiarism, recycling, and text recycling are terms used to describe forms of plagiarism where authors copy their own works, representing them with minor changes without citation to their own previous publications. Duplication, another synonym, may refer to plagiarism or self-plagiarism related to the republication of entire articles. A redundant publication is work multiply published in part or in its entirety (in the same or another language) without justification and without reference to the original source. Depending on the extent of the material copied, the originality of the material copied, and citations to the original source, plagiarism may be classified as research misconduct or questionable practice. Plagiarism checks can be carried out using artificial intelligence, and since automated checks have been implemented by journals, it has become a common reason for article retraction. *Also see* **Citation** and **FFP**.

Policy: A guideline or set of rules of an organization. *Also see* **Procedure** and **Regulation**.

Post-publication peer review: *See* **Peer review** and **Sleuthing**.

Power : The ability to influence others. In the academic setting, role asymmetry permits seniors to influence junior colleagues. The power imbalance between research colleagues may be abused in coercive citations, unethical authorship, and other irresponsible research and publication practices. In Global North–South research collaborations, researchers from institutions in developed countries enjoy asymmetrically more resources, prestige, and influence over their less developed country partners, opening the door to the possibility of authorship abuse. In biomedical research, the personal authority that healthcare professionals exercise over vulnerable patients can sometimes lead to abuse, e.g., manipulation of research consent procedures. It is the responsibility of healthcare professionals to ensure that patients are never forced to enter into studies as participants. Consent for participation should be fully informed and entirely voluntary. *Also see* **Participants, Ethics dumping, Parachute research, Colonization of research, Coercive citation practices**, and **Authorship abuse**.

Preprint: A publicly posted draft version of a scientific manuscript prior to completion of its formal peer review. It is usually simultaneously posted at the first submission of a manuscript to a journal. It offers the opportunity for public comment (pre-review) alongside formal peer review organized by the journal. Preprints are not considered prior publication, so they are not disqualifiers for submission to a journal. Preprints usually have DOIs (digital object identifiers) and can be cited like any other paper. The preprint version is updated with a link to the final published version. *Also see* **Open science, Version of record, Open access publication**, and **Peer review**.

Principle: A moral value and concept, i.e., something that distinguishes between right and wrong, for guiding researchers' behavior. *Also see* **Standard, Ethics**, and **Moral values**.

Procedure: Step-by-step instructions for implementing a policy in an organization. *Also see* **Policy** and **Regulation**.

Professional regulatory body: By law, healthcare professionals must be registered with a professional regulatory body to ensure they are fit and licensed to practice. Regulated healthcare professionals are many, including but not limited to biomedical scientists, chiropractors, clinical scientists, dentists, dental nurses and technicians, dietitians, doctors, hearing aid dispensers, midwives, nurses, nursing associates, occupational therapists, operating department practitioners, opticians, osteopaths, paramedics, pharmacists, physiotherapists, radiographers, speech and language therapists, etc. (in alphabetical order). A regulatory body may undertake a fitness-to-practice investigation upon being alerted about a research integrity concern. The term professional regulatory body should not be confused with the term regulator used in other contexts in this book, e.g., a formal body set up for official approvals of medicines and devices, e.g., European Medicines Agency (EMA). *Also see* **Regulator of drugs and devices** and **Securities regulator**.

Professional Societies: *See* **Societies**.

Proof-of-concept study: A term used to describe a study conducted as an early translational step to inform "go/no-go" decisions about proceeding with further research. It ranks low in the evidence-based medicine hierarchy. *Also see* **Research translation**.

Prospective registration: Pre-registration of a research project in a publicly available registry before the enrollment of the first participant. *Also see* **Research transparency**.

Publication asymmetry: The imbalance in publishing where original research is readily accepted and amplified in high-prestige journals, while criticisms, replications, or corrections remain invisible in low-profile journals. This creates a bias favoring initial claims (even if flawed) over challenges. *Also see* **Halo effect**.

Publication process manipulation: A form of research misconduct in the publication process. It may involve authors as well as reviewers. Examples include organization of or taking part in fake peer review, unauthorized use of information gained through peer reviewing activities, confidentiality violation through disclosure of peer-reviewed information to others, and coercive citation practices. *Also see* **Coercive citation practices** and **CiteScore**.

Publish or perish: An academic culture in which research organizations value the number of papers rather than their integrity, quality, or impact. *Also see* **DORA**, **CoARA**, and **SCOPE**.

Publish then perish: If misconduct allegations are investigated and errors found, the publication may figuratively perish with its retraction. With massive retractions, entire journals may disappear from listings or perish altogether as entities. *Also see* **Retraction**.

Publisher: An organization or entity whose business is to prepare and issue works, such as books, magazines, journals, etc., for public distribution. Publishers are responsible for managing the editorial process, evaluating the submissions received, ensuring publication quality, making content available to readers, and investigating publication integrity concerns raised. *Also see* **Journal**.

PubMed: Freely available interface of the general biomedical research database Medline, which contains publication records with and without abstracts from 1966 onwards (ncbi .nlm.nih.gov/PubMed). It covers around 5,200 journals, whereas it is estimated that there are 16,000 biomedical journals.

PubPeer: An online platform for post-publication peer review (pubpeer.com). *Also see* **Sleuthing**, **Peer review**, and **Open peer review**.

Questionable research practices (QRPs): Irresponsible research and publication practices that are regarded as unethical or unprofessional but fall short of being included in the definition of research misconduct. There are many QRPs, including but not limited to selective outcome reporting, the introduction of spin in the description of research findings, various forms of publication process manipulation, etc. *Also see* **Research misconduct**.

Randomized clinical trial: A clinical trial involving random allocation of eligible, consenting human participants to arms or intervention groups and their follow-up to compare group outcomes. The random allocation is kept concealed from both trialists and participants until eligibility assessments have been performed and informed consent has been obtained. This type of trial is launched after pre-clinical and proof-of-concept studies have established the underlying mechanisms and the plausibility by which the intervention could have an effect on the target condition and have shown it to be likely safe and tolerable. *Also see* **Clinical trial** and **Systematic review**.

Recklessness: Indifference or disregard toward the risk of potentially false information being produced from research undertaken without exercising proper care or caution. *Also see* **Research misconduct**.

Redundant publication: *See* **Plagiarism**.

Regulations: The directives that an authority creates, maintains, and enforces by law. *Also see* **Policy**, **Procedure**, and **Regulator of drugs and devices**.

Regulator of drugs and devices: A formal body set up for official approvals of medicines and devices, e.g., European Medicines Agency (EMA), US Food and Drug Administration (FDA), UK Medicines and Health care products Regulatory Agency (MHRA), Health Canada, etc. *Also see* **Regulations** and **Professional regulatory body**.

Research culture: The academic environment comprising of the norms, values, expectations, attitudes, and behaviors within research organizations. It strongly influences research integrity. For example, the publish or perish culture is believed to be associated with authorship abuse and other forms of misconduct. Academic freedom, collegiality, collaboration, equality and diversity, ethics and professionalism, openness, accountability, and transparency are all features of the research culture. *Also see* **Publish or perish**, **Research integrity**, **Research transparency**, and **Open science**.

Research Ethics Committee (REC): *See* **Human Research Ethics Committee**.

Research governance: The system set up by institutions to oversee the conduct of research under their auspices. Governance approvals for studies and oversight of their compliance with ethical and professional standards are enforced through audits undertaken according to the established institutional research policies and procedures. *Also see* **Human Research Ethics Committee**, **Sponsor**, **Research integrity**, **Audit**, and **Research ethics**.

Research integrity: Undertaking research in accordance with ethical and professional principles and standards. Integrity failures may result from honest or innocent errors as well as from intentional, knowing, or reckless research misconduct. *Also see* **Research misconduct** and **Questionable research practices**.

Research misconduct: Unethical or unprofessional conduct in research and publication that is intentional, knowing, or reckless, i.e., negligent. In some definitions, misconduct is limited to fabrication, falsification, or plagiarism (FFP), and in others, unethical authorship or authorship abuse, conflict of interest mismanagement, publication process manipulation, and misconduct related to misconduct investigation procedures, etc., are also included. Many questionable research practices do not make it into the definition of misconduct. Honest error is not misconduct. *Also see* **Questionable research practices**.

Research translation: Moving from the bench to the bedside, i.e., from theoretical research knowledge about disease mechanisms gained in the laboratory (basic research), all the way to its application into routine clinical practice and healthcare decision-making (applied research). Clinical trials, particularly randomized clinical trials and their evidence syntheses, are key translational steps leading to improved health. *Also see* **Clinical trials**, **Basic research**, and **Applied research**.

Research transparency: Transparency in research includes open science practices such as prospective registration, protocol publication, *a priori* statistical analysis plan, data sharing, timely and complete public reporting, conflict of interest disclosure, open research assessment, open publication practice, etc. *Also see* **Open science**.

ResearchGate: Primarily a professional networking service for scientists, it hosts self-archived content, including conference proceedings, abstracts, preprints, presentation slides, posters, and papers uploaded by scientists themselves. It also calculates some metrics like the RG Score based on scientific activity and content, which may include citations from other indexed sources. ResearchGate is a popular means for gaining visibility rapidly.

Respondent in a research misconduct investigation: The researcher whose research conduct is the subject of a complaint or is being investigated formally by their employer, funder, journal, professional regulatory body, or the law court. *Also see* **Complaint**, **Questionable research practice**, **Research integrity**, **Research misconduct**, and **Professional regulatory body**.

Responsible research conduct: Research conduct that is compliant with ethical and professional principles and standards. *Also see* **Research integrity**, **Research misconduct**, and **Questionable research practices**.

Retraction: Withdrawal or removal of a published paper from the research record because of a variety of reasons, including the discovery of a flaw in its integrity, e.g., a post-publication reassessment showing that the data or results reported have major errors. A research misconduct investigation may have established that the paper in question harbored research misconduct or perhaps there was an honest error. Journals publish retraction notices and identify retracted papers in electronic databases with reasons for retraction, which are not always clearly stated. In case of honest errors, journals may retract and republish a paper or may publish a corrigendum. *Also see* **Expression of concern**, **Erratum**, **Corrigendum**, **Research misconduct**, and **Questionable research practices**.

Retraction Watch: A project of the Center for Scientific Integrity (centerforscientificintegrity.org), it is a blog dedicated to reporting on research misconduct and tracking journal article retractions (retractionwatch.com). *Also see* **Sleuthing**.

RIAT: An international initiative to address the problem of unpublished and misreported (inaccurate or incomplete) trials (Restoring Invisible and Abandoned Trials, restoringtrials.org). *Also see* **AllTrials**.

Ripple effect: A situation in which an initial event triggers a series of consequences that affect increasingly distant parts of the ecosystem, just as dropping a stone into a pond creates circular waves that move away from the center, reaching areas not directly impacted in the first contact. In the context of the retraction of a scientific article, the ripple effect refers to how the retraction triggers a cascade of negative consequences that extend far beyond the retracted study, e.g., contamination of evidence as the retracted study continues to be cited, collateral damage to the "innocent" co-authors whose ability to obtain funding or enter new collaborations is potentially reduced, many retracted authors leave academic employment, institutions may suffer loss of funding or they may be fined, journals' reputations may suffer or they may even close down after massive retractions, among other outcomes.

Scientific sleuthing: *See* **Sleuthing**.

Scientific virtue: A character trait or a disposition to consistently act in a manner that will best achieve research excellence. Intellectual honesty, accountability, meticulousness, transparency, and other related virtues are essential to research integrity and responsible research conduct. *Also see* **Accountability**, **Intellectual honesty**, **Research integrity**, and **Research misconduct**.

SCOPE: A framework for evaluating research responsibly produced by INORMS, the International Network of Research Management Societies (Start with what is valued, Context considerations, Options for evaluating, Probe deeply, and Evaluate the evaluation; DOI: 10.26188/21919527.v1). *Also see* **Publish or perish**, **CoARA**, and **DORA**.

Scopus: A global abstract and citation database of scientific literature, owned by Elsevier. It has a content selection and advisory board. It indexes over 25,000 journals and produces the CiteScore to rank journals. The *h*-index produced by Scopus tends to be intermediate between that obtained via Web of Science or Google Scholar. *Also see* ***h*-index**, **Web of Science**, and **Google Scholar**.

Securities regulator: A formal body or agency set up by the government for independent oversight in financial markets, such as stock exchanges and trading, to protect investors and ensure fair, transparent, and stable operations. *Also see* **Regulator of drugs and devices** and **Professional regulatory body**.

Security: Refers to a multitude of tradable financial instruments, such as stocks, bonds, investment contracts, etc., that are sold to investors by corporations and governments to raise capital. *Also see* **Initial public offering (IPO)**.

Selective outcome reporting: A difference in the outcomes reported in a published studies compared to its original ethics committee approved protocol and prospective registration. The prospective registration requirements implemented since 2005 have encouraged reporting of the result for the original primary outcome, even if it shows a statistically non-significant result on study completion. In the past, if the original primary outcome showed a statistically non-significant result on study completion, there used to be a tendency to report statistically significant results of non-primary outcomes. There may be an element of p-hacking involved even when the primary outcome cannot be easily changed, and that is why an *a priori* statistical analysis plan is required. *Also see* **p-hacking** and **Prospective registration**.

Selective reporting: *See* **Selective outcome reporting**.

Self-plagiarism: *See* **Plagiarism**.

Shanghai Ranking: Also known as the Shanghai Ranking, the Academic Ranking of World Universities is one of the most influential global research-based university rankings. It incorporates: alumni and faculty Nobel Prizes and Fields Medals (a third); highly cited researchers (a fifth); papers in top journals (a fifth); *Science* and *Nature* papers (a fifth); and total research output (a tenth). Retractions may indirectly, not directly, affect the ranking. After giving the first 100 ranks individually, it groups universities in bands, e.g., 401–500, to reflect methodological imprecision.

Sleuthing: Investigation of research and publication integrity concerns by independent researchers who do not have a formal role. Sleuthing typically involves post-publication investigation of possible research and publication misconduct and questionable research practices by volunteer researchers. Data sleuths tend to report their findings via blogging, social media, and online platforms such as PubPeer (pubpeer.com), Retraction Watch (retractionwatch.com), and For Better Science (forbetterscience.com), among others. Sleuthing involves the use of validated (e.g., digital image forensics, plagiarism checks) as well as so far unvalidated instruments to signpost the possibility of research integrity flaws. Sleuthing may be considered an informal investigation that can provide the underpinning evidence for making a formal complaint or for evaluation in a formal research misconduct investigation. It is not regulated by professional codes in the same way as a journalistic investigation. *Also see* **Peer review**, **Whistleblower**, **Complaint**, **Journalistic investigation**, **Questionable research practice**, **Research integrity**, and **Research misconduct**.

Societies: Non-profit organizations (associations or bodies) that seek to further a particular healthcare profession and the interests of their patients. Societies are made up of a membership of healthcare professionals. Societies tend to have an official journal, a committee for developing clinical practice guidelines, an annual conference with posters, oral presentations, and workshops, etc. Members of professional societies may participate in planning and conducting clinical studies in their specialty. As professionals, they have a seat at the table in determining priorities alongside other stakeholders such as patients, caregivers, and public representatives. *Also see* **Institution**, **Funder**, and **Journal**.

Spin: Exaggerating the implications or importance of research findings in order to increase the likelihood of publication. It is a questionable research practice that distorts the interpretation or extrapolation of research findings, leading to a mismatch between conclusions drawn and results observed, e.g., attribution of causality in the absence of an appropriate study design, recommending an intervention more or less strongly than that underpinned by the observed changes in outcomes, claiming equivalence in a statistically non-significant result, prioritizing per protocol rather than intention to treat analysis, discrediting evidence of association (reverse spin), etc. A partial retraction may be required to correct the version of record that contains spin. *Also see* **Questionable research practice**, **Research integrity**, and **Research misconduct**.

Spin-off company: *See* **Spinout company**.

Spinout company: Also known as a spin-off, it is a new, independent business entity formed from a university (or a large business) to commercialize specific technology or research to leverage the parent organization's knowledge. *Also see* **Security**.

Sponsor: Clinical trial regulations require that a sponsor makes proper arrangements to initiate and conduct trials. For researchers employed in an academic setting, it is usually their own institution that acts as the sponsor. In commercial clinical trials seeking regulatory approval of a drug, the sponsor may be a pharmaceutical company. *Also see* **Institution** and **Regulator of drugs and devices**.

Standard: Specification of the behavior that must be adhered to when planning, conducting, analyzing, and reporting a research study. *Also see* **Principle**, **GCP**, **Ethics**, and **Moral values**.

Statistical analysis plan : Development of the analysis outlined in a study registration and protocol into a detailed *a priori* statistical analysis plan of the primary outcome, the secondary outcomes and other variables before the dataset is closed and prepared for formal analysis. The database is locked following the collection of the outcome data from the last recruited participant. Not included among the 14 terms in the contributor roles taxonomy, preparation of the statistical analysis plan should be a recognized role in a publication. *Also see* **CRediT**, **p-hacking**, and **Selective outcome reporting**.

Subjects: *See* **Participants**.

Systematic review : An evidence synthesis type that summarizes the evidence on a clearly formulated question, either narrow or broad, using systematic and explicit methods to identify, select, and appraise relevant primary studies, and to extract, collate, and report their findings. It may or may not use statistical meta-analysis. *Also see* **Guideline**.

TOP: Guidelines for Transparency and Openness Promotion (TOP) in journal policies and practices (osf.io/ud578). *Also see* **Journal** and **Research transparency**.

Transparency: *See* **Research transparency**.

Transparency in research misconduct investigation: The requirement that steps of a research misconduct investigation are clearly laid out to the respondent, who has the right to be informed about the process and the stage of the procedure at any time during the investigation. *Also see* **Respondent**.

Unethical authorship: *See* **Authorship abuse**.

Version of record: The final published version of an article (following the manuscript's peer review, editorial assessments, and author revisions) in its definitive form with copyediting and typesetting completed, metadata applied, and DOI (digital object identifier) allocated. It may appear as an online accepted manuscript before the release of the version of record. Depending on the copyright agreement, the version of record may be immediately open access, or there may be an embargo period. *Also see* **Open science**, **Open access publication**, **Preprint**, and **Peer review**.

WAME: World Association of Medical Editors. Among other things, it aims to improve editorial standards and promote professionalism in medical editing through education, self-criticism, and self-regulation (wame.org). *Also see* **Journal**, **ICMJE**, and **COPE**.

Web of Science (WoS): A global citation database of science, owned by Clarivate. It includes journals that meet its quality and integrity standards. It indexes around 20,000 journals and issues the "official" impact factor to rank journals. If a journal is not in the WoS collection, it cannot have an "official" impact factor. The WoS *h*-index tends to be more conservative than that obtained via Scopus or Google Scholar. *Also see* ***h*-index**, **Scopus**, and **Google Scholar**.

Whistleblower: An individual, also known as the complainant, who reports a possible current or past breach of research integrity, making an allegation of research misconduct or questionable research practice. Complaints ought to be made in good faith with reasonable belief or evidence of wrongdoing. The complaint made may be found or there may be no case to answer on investigation. *Also see* **Sleuthing**, **GCP**, **Questionable research practice**, **Research integrity**, and **Research misconduct**.

WoS: *See* **Web of Science**.

References

This book focuses on core information about health research integrity and on learning lessons through publicly available investigations of allegations of research misconduct and questionable practices. Its evidence sources are listed within each chapter. The following works and discussions with colleagues who collectively have expertise in health research have helped shape its discourse:

- International multi-stakeholder consensus statement on patient, carer and public involvement to enhance clinical trial integrity. *Account Res* 2026. DOI: 10.1080/08989621.2026.2647346.
- International multistakeholder consensus statement on post-publication integrity issues in randomized clinical trials by Cairo Consensus Group. *Int J Gynaecol Obstet* 2025;169:1093–1115. DOI: 10.1002/ijgo.16118.
- Ethics and informed consent in clinical trial integrity: An international, multi-stakeholder consensus statement by Cairo Consensus Group. *Int J Gynaecol Obstet* 2026;172:828–844. DOI: 10.1002/ijgo.70374.
- International multi-stakeholder consensus statement on clinical trial integrity. *BJOG* 2023;130:1096–1111. DOI: 10.1111/1471-0528.17451.
- Integrity of randomized clinical trials: Performance of integrity tests and checklists requires assessment. *Int J Gynaecol Obstet* 2023;163:733-743. DOI: 10.1002/ijgo.14837.
- *Integrity of Randomized Clinical Trials: How to Prevent Research Misconduct and Ensure Transparency*. London: Taylor & Francis Publishing, 2024. DOI: 10.1201/9781003461401.

There is a need for harmonization of definitions for the various stakeholders to speak the same language, so the book provides a detailed glossary of terms. The sources of definitions consulted are listed below:

- Glossary. *Integrity of Randomized Clinical Trials: How to Prevent Research Misconduct and Ensure Transparency*. London: Taylor & Francis Publishing, 2024:162–193. DOI: 10.1201/9781003461401.
- Glossary. *Systematic Reviews to Support Evidence-Based Medicine. How to Appraise, Conduct and Publish Reviews*. 3rd Edition. London: Taylor & Francis Publishing, 2022:193–206. DOI: 10.1201/9781003220039.
- Glossary for Research and Academic Ethics and Integrity. URL: https://h2020integrity.eu/resources/glossary.

Index

For Product Safety Concerns and Information please contact our EU representative GPSR@taylorandfrancis.com
Taylor & Francis Verlag GmbH, Kaufingerstraße 24, 80331 München, Germany

www.ingramcontent.com/pod-product-compliance
Lightning Source LLC
LaVergne TN
LVHW010631190926
848399LV00033B/305

* 9 7 8 1 0 4 1 1 0 6 0 2 9 *